THE
Men'sHealth®
COVER
MODEL
WORKOUT

THE
Men'sHealth®
COVER MODEL
WORKOUT

BODY-SCULPTING SECRETS OF THE WORLD'S TOP FITNESS MODEL

BY
OWEN McKIBBIN

WITH KELLY GARRETT

RODALE

Book design by Megan Clayton

Library of Congress Cataloging-in-Publication Data
McKibbin, Owen.
The men's health cover model workout : body-sculpting secrets of the world's top fitness model /
by Owen McKibbin with Kelly Garrett.
p.   cm.
Includes index.
ISBN 1-57954-744-3 hardcover
1. Bodybuilding.   2. Physical fitness.   3. Exercise.   4. Male models.   I. Title: Body-sculpting
secrets of the world's top fitness model.   II. Garrett, Kelly.   III. Title.
GV546.5M393   2003
646.7'5—dc21   2002154810

Distributed to the book trade by St. Martin's Press

2 4 6 8 10 9 7 5 3 1   hardcover

Visit us on the Web at www.menshealthbooks.com, or call us toll-free at (800) 848-4735.

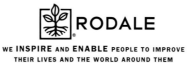

RODALE
WE INSPIRE AND ENABLE PEOPLE TO IMPROVE
THEIR LIVES AND THE WORLD AROUND THEM

I dedicate this book
to those enlightened individuals
who inspire, give life, and create.

Mom,
for showing me what
true strength and perseverance
are all about.

Lisa,
for showing me that love
at first sight is not a myth,
for giving me strength
in the face of adversity,
and for being my beautiful wife
and best friend.

Blaze,
for restoring my belief
in mankind's purity and goodness.
You fill my soul with love every day.
I'm so proud to be your father.

Dad,
for always watching over me
and my family,
from heaven.

My love for you is infinite.

CONTENTS

ACKNOWLEDGMENTS

Many people besides me had a major hand in the creation of this book.

• First and foremost, the staff of *Men's Health* magazine and Rodale: David Zinczenko, who blessed me with the privilege of representing the magazine and, more important, who cares about my family; George Karabotsos, who always takes my calls and lets me break his balls, even when he has deadlines to meet; Lou Schuler, who opened my mind and made this a better book; Kelly Garrett, who made sense of my chicken scratch and transformed my thoughts into an actual book; Charlene Lutz, Adam Campbell, Jeremy Katz, Karen Mazzotta, Aimee Geller Promisel, Stephen Perrine, Susan Eugster, and so many others who have always put forth great efforts in facilitating my career.

• The wonderful people at *Extra* TV provided me the platform and opportunity to reach the masses with my fitness philosophy and methods. Their unrelenting trust and support helped build AskOwen.com into a Web site visited by millions.

• The people at *CBS News*, *48 Hours*, and *The New York Times*, whose excellence in reporting is unparalleled.

• The countless agents, photographers, stylists, and makeup artists, with their professionalism and meticulous attention to detail.

I thank you all profoundly for your efforts and for your interest in me and my career.

I
WASN'T
BORN
THIS WAY

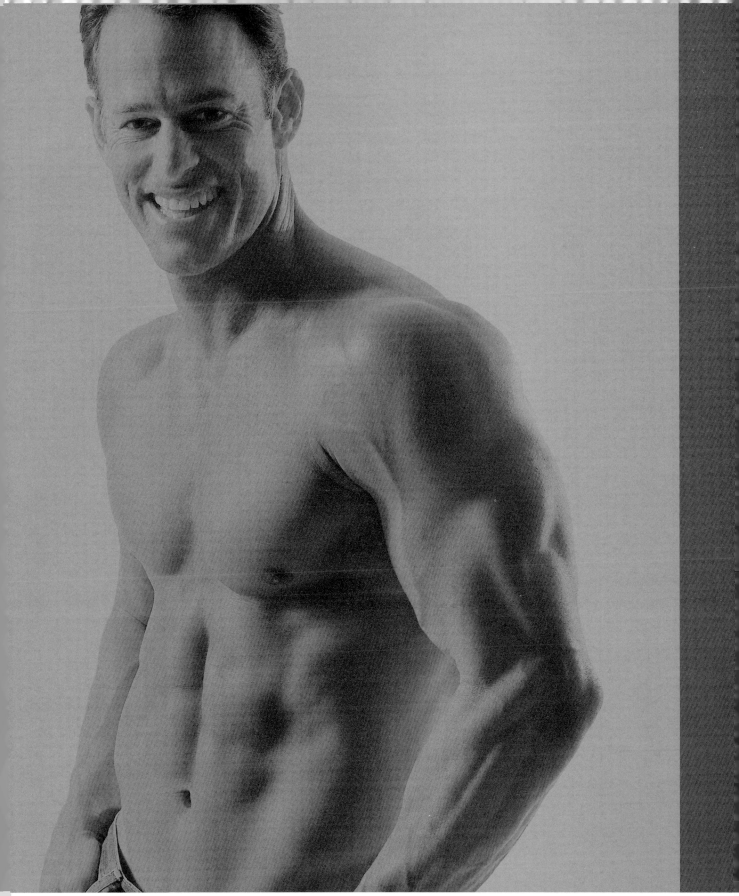

Men's

BOOST YOUR
SEX AP
50 Ways to Do It, F

WANT MUS
EAT THIS (p.7

FREE POSTER

GET
STRO
This Guy's →
Ultimate Secre

STRIP AW
STRESS

YOUR
PERFE
WEIGH
Get there, s

THE PROMISE

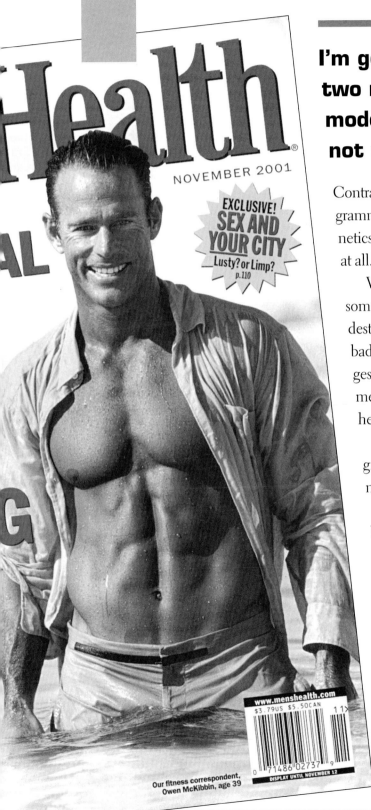

I'm going to let you in on the two real secrets to a cover model body. I guarantee they're not what you'd expect.

Contrary to popular belief, I wasn't genetically programmed to be the *Men's Health* cover guy. In fact, if genetics had its way, you'd never find me in *Men's Health* at all. Or in any other magazine, for that matter.

Where you'd probably find me is lazing on a beach somewhere—a shaggy, obese loser with terrible teeth, destroyed knees, bum ankles, a broken spine, and a bad reputation. You'd find a smoker with a habit of ingesting enormous quantities of beer and other self-medications to blunt the pain long enough for a heart attack to claim him before middle age does.

Why? Because my body wasn't genetically programmed to look good for the camera. It was genetically programmed to hurt like hell.

Doctors said I had the knees of a 50-year-old by the time I was 10. The anterior cruciate ligament (ACL) that so many athletes worry about wasn't ever a problem for my left knee. I simply never had one.

A broken spine tortured me for my entire college and pro beach volleyball career. It may have been congenital.

I wore braces until I was 28.

Obesity plagues my family. Two of my siblings are extremely overweight. Until recently, everyone in my family smoked except me.

Heart disease is in my bloodline. My oldest brother has had two heart attacks. My mom had her own heart attack. My dad died from his heart attack before he could celebrate his 42nd birthday.

That's the genetic hand I was dealt. None of the cards was the "king of covers." I slipped that one in myself.

My ace in the hole was a determination to keep myself stronger and fitter than anybody who dared to compete with me. No matter what else was going on with my body (and believe me, *a lot* else was going on with my body), I never strayed from my commitment to stay in the best shape I possibly could.

Because of that, I enjoyed an improbable run of 8 years as a pretty damn good athlete in what was really my second-best sport. That success, in turn, was the launching pad for my career in the modeling game.

But it got even better. Every man has a turning point in his life, one of those defining moments when, for better or worse, he shifts gears and makes some kind of radical turn onto a new road. Mine came in 1994 at the age of 31. And it was definitely a turn for the better. It involved a surgical team, a promise, and a girl.

I'll let you in on the details later. For now, I'll just say that my 1994 epiphany gave me what I needed to take things to the next level. I worked out even harder—and smarter. More important, I expanded my understanding of what it really means to lead a healthy life. It was then—and only then—that I was ready to do the kind of body shots worthy of *Men's Health*. And that's exactly what I did.

The bottom line is this: It wasn't genetics that landed me on the cover of *Men's Health*. It wasn't even hard work, though there was plenty of that. It was the *motivation* to do the hard work in the first place. And it was the *discipline* to stick with it no matter what. Everything else followed from those two things.

Motivation and discipline aren't genetic traits. And they're not my exclusive domain, by any means. They're inside *you*, ready to go to work. They're your ticket to a great body and healthy life, just as they were mine.

I'm going to give you a lot of specific advice in the pages ahead. I'm going to tell you my training secrets. I'm going to lay out some detailed strength and endurance programs. I'm going to suggest what kind of foods you should be eating and when you should be eating them. I'm going to show you how to do things my way. At the same time I'm going to help you find ways of doing them that are right for you.

But none of those specifics is half as important as the lesson in determination that my path represents. If you ignore every shred of specific information I give you in the Cover Model Workout and still come away with the motivation and discipline to get your body into the kind of

> "Every man has a turning point in his life, one of those defining moments when, for better or worse, he shifts gears and makes some kind of radical turn onto a new road."

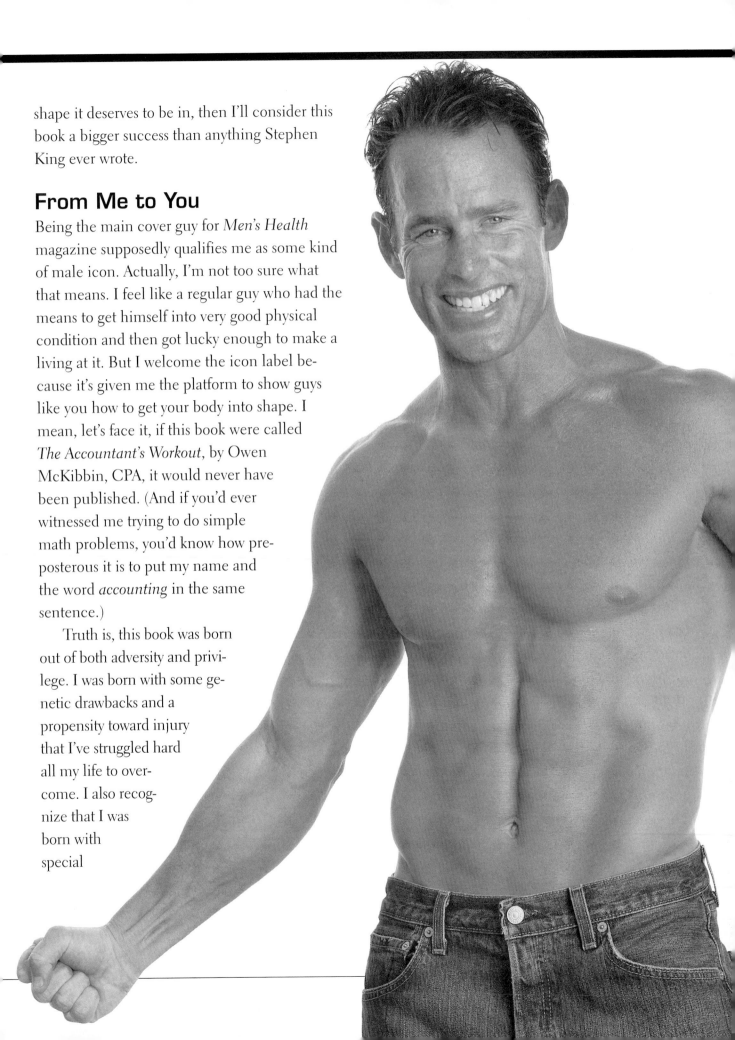

shape it deserves to be in, then I'll consider this book a bigger success than anything Stephen King ever wrote.

From Me to You

Being the main cover guy for *Men's Health* magazine supposedly qualifies me as some kind of male icon. Actually, I'm not too sure what that means. I feel like a regular guy who had the means to get himself into very good physical condition and then got lucky enough to make a living at it. But I welcome the icon label because it's given me the platform to show guys like you how to get your body into shape. I mean, let's face it, if this book were called *The Accountant's Workout*, by Owen McKibbin, CPA, it would never have been published. (And if you'd ever witnessed me trying to do simple math problems, you'd know how preposterous it is to put my name and the word *accounting* in the same sentence.)

Truth is, this book was born out of both adversity and privilege. I was born with some genetic drawbacks and a propensity toward injury that I've struggled hard all my life to overcome. I also recognize that I was born with special athletic ability and some mysterious light-reflecting quality that cameras seem to like. The important thing is that by focusing on my own physical fitness, I've been able to minimize the damage of my negative inheritance and maximize the potential of my positive inheritance.

Along the way, I learned a lot about the best ways to exercise. I learned what works and what doesn't. I learned what it means to eat right. And I learned how to use a tough, no-excuses-allowed mental approach to get the job done. I didn't master those things because I'm smart. I mastered them because circumstances determined that physical fitness would be my life's pursuit.

Now I want to share my knowledge with you.

This book is called *The* Men's Health *Cover Model Workout* because it's based on the programs I've developed to keep myself in the kind of shape necessary to appear on *Men's Health* covers. But don't take the title too literally. Most guys won't be candidates for cover modeling, or any kind of modeling. (There's that mysterious light-reflecting quality I mentioned; you either have it or you don't.) Which is fine, since most guys don't have the slightest desire to be models.

But every guy is a candidate to get his body into the best shape it can possibly be in—which is the shape it's *supposed* to be in. Cover model fitness is a metaphor for that kind of top-notch superfitness. Think of it as the fitness level you'd want to see reflected on the cover of your autobiography.

The Life You Deserve

What the fitness program in this book will achieve for you is nothing less than a better life. Every single aspect of your existence—your

health, your self-confidence, your family life, even your employment prospects—improves as a direct result of getting yourself into peak shape, the kind of condition you didn't know you were capable of achieving. And peak shape comes from nothing more than letting your body do what it was designed to do: move.

Five thousand years ago, if you weren't willing to get out there and run and jump and throw spears, you'd starve to death. The human body hasn't changed all that much since then, but now we can get all the food we want without leaving the couch. I'm all for convenience, but if we want to do right by our

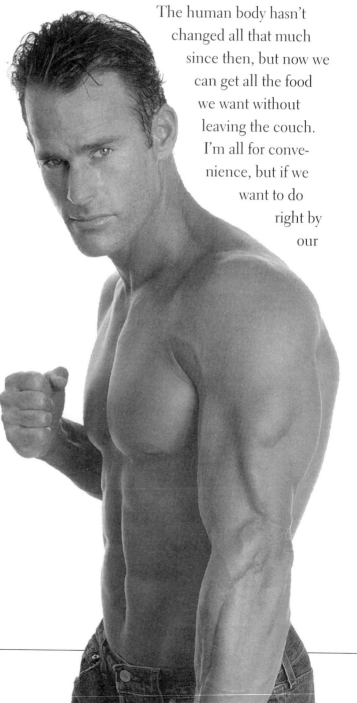

bodies, we have to find an alternative way to get our asses in gear every day. That's what exercise is.

The most amazing thing about exercise is that the physical and mental benefits start showing up *as you do it.* Those of you who are coming to the Cover Model Workout to get even better already know this, but for the newbies out there, I've got some great news. You don't have to wait until your biceps bulge. As soon as you get yourself into the habit of working out every day, you're going to start noticing changes in your head, even before you start seeing them in the mirror.

For example, when I'm working out I'm in "beast mode," and there's nothing that I can't run through or over. But afterward, you have to check me for a pulse. Why? Because I feel cleansed. Not just tired, but calm. Balanced. *At peace.*

You're going to feel that too—sooner rather than later. The real-life benefits are immediately tangible. You feel good about yourself again. Your coping capacity zooms. It's still no fun to be stuck in traffic, but you deal with it a lot better with a workout under your belt. From now on, you're going to spend a lot less time being pissed off.

Keep with the program for a while and your body starts feeling the benefits too. Lean muscle mass begins to replace body fat. That in turn jacks up your metabolism so you burn more fat all day long. Your bones are denser, your connective tissues thicker and healthier. Your sugar levels even out and you stop craving junk food. You don't feel bloated all the time. Your circulation and heart rate improve. Your mood is better

"Every guy is a candidate to get his body into the best shape it can possibly be in—which is the shape it's supposed to be in."

and your pants are looser. You can walk up a flight of stairs and still be able to talk when you get to the top. There's a spring in your step and an energy supply that won't quit. You're on fire.

Then you start *seeing* the benefits. You look in the mirror and find good things there for a change: the set of your shoulders, the way your clothes fit, the new tone in your legs, some muscle definition where flab once reigned, maybe a little ab muscle starting to show. They're little things with huge implications for the quality of your life.

They're what the Cover Model Workout is all about.

You, Meeting Every Challenge

Exercise leads to health and strength. But there's another reward in the form of a powerful tool for taking on challenges and leading a life of achievement. That tool is called self-esteem, and it empowers you to do anything.

In my first year on the Pro Beach Volleyball Tour (yes, I was a professional beach volleyball player, but more on that later), I remember watching superstars like Karch Kiraly and Tim Hovland slamming balls straight down over the net during warmup like they were shooting cannons down an elevator shaft. My technique was nowhere near as good as theirs.

I knew I'd done my homework. I knew I was mentally and physically strong enough as a result of my training to compete with these guys. And you know what? I won my fair share of matches.

That's what pumped-up self-esteem from regular exercise did for me on the sand. It's done the same for me in my modeling career and in my acting career—and everything else in my life.

It's going to do the same for you. As you work your way through the programs in this book, your self-esteem is going to come together and solidify like a new planet. You're going to get in great shape, and you're going to win your fair share of life's challenges. You may lose some too, but you're never again going to wonder if you belong in the game.

> "As you work your way through the programs in this book, your self-esteem is going to come together and solidify like a new planet."

Presumed Guilty: The Burdens of Being Buff

Another perk of my so-called male icon status is the opportunity to put down misconceptions and negative attitudes that some people harbor about guys who work at getting their bodies into top shape. Most people are pretty much aware that a lean, muscled male body is a healthier male body. But that doesn't stop a lot of them from impugning your motives or questioning your methods.

Listen to some of the stuff I get all the time. If things go right, it may be aimed your way in the near future.

"He's not that great. . . ." I'm scrutinized all the time by people who've never laid eyes on me in the flesh. *Men's Health* gets swamped with letters from people insisting that this photo must have been airbrushed or that photo was doctored because his abs can't pos-

sibly look like that, or such and such a pose was obviously faked. They're wrong, but they're avid about it.

In person, the scrutiny is more intense. As soon as my shirt goes off on a hot day, I can feel the eyes boring in and the brain neurons computing the visual information. If people are worked up enough to try to bring me down, I must be doing something right.

"What he's really pumping is ego. . . ." Get vaccinated for your health, and they call you smart. Lift weights for the same reason, and they call you self-absorbed. Go figure.

The inflated-ego stereotype comes from the basic misconception that vanity is what drives a man to develop his body to its maximum potential. But what's really doing the driving, in my opinion, is self-respect.

This book is *not* about vanity. It's not even about looks. And if that sounds strange coming from a muscle model, keep reading. We're not doing a salon-style male-makeover here. We're on a much deeper voyage. People work like dogs to save for retirement, and no one thinks that's vanity. But if you work out a few hours a week in the gym so that you live long enough to retire, that's vanity? I don't get it.

"What an airhead. . . ." The stereotype that hunks are slower than a one-rep max is as old as history and still going strong. People assume that a really fit guy is some kind of male bimbo trading on superficial appearance because he's got nothing else in his tool kit.

What they're saying, basically, is that smart guys are ineligible to develop their bodies past a certain point. That to me is a much dumber statement than anything we male bimbos could ever come up with. Anyone who believes such a thing should talk to some of my fellow fitness models and see if his prejudices hold up. What he'll find is that some will impress him with their intelligence, some will come off as average thinkers, and some won't measure up to his standards. (By the way, they'll all be in better shape than he is.)

"He looks like a bully. . . ." I won't be throwing a lot of scientific data at you in the pages ahead, but I guarantee that no study has ever found any correlation between muscle size and character flaws. That doesn't keep some people from assuming any dude with a well-developed torso must be a brute who can only use physical intimidation against those smaller than him to get his way. They must have come to this conclusion by watching Popeye cartoons, because real life doesn't bear it out.

I will say this, however. Even though I'm not one to throw my weight around, I'm capable of uncorking some serious testosterone when challenged on the playing field or the basketball court. Life poses occasional physical challenges. There's nothing wrong with being up for them.

"He must be doing something really

extreme. . . ." I plead guilty to this one, with an explanation.

First of all, you don't need to be extreme, per se, to get yourself into top shape. But you do need to be extremely consistent. You need to work hard at least five or six times a week. That said, I'm probably more extreme in my workouts than most guys. For example, my idea of fitness running isn't a paced 5-mile jog. It's 20 minutes of intense wind sprints up The Hill, a viciously inclined street in the foothills of Santa Monica. Or it's 10 sets on a public stairway in Santa Monica Canyon that's affectionately called The Stairs— each set consisting of taking the 172 steps two at a time, with 15 pullups after each one.

I sneak in workouts whenever and wherever I can—in a hotel stairwell or on the way to the Department of Motor Vehicles. And I hate taking days off. If I have to take a day off, I feel as if I'd been beaten with a stick. Is that too extreme? For most people, maybe. But not for me. Extreme is a relative term. My extreme ways are the result of the motivation I recruited and the determination I developed to deal with the obstacles I had to overcome to get into shape in the first place.

Also, I'm a pro. I stay fit for a living. I have to be cover-ready on short notice. Those are extreme requirements, and they call for extreme measures.

I've designed the Cover Model Workout with enough flexibility that you can take it to whatever extreme you see fit. The harder you work, the fitter you get. What matters most, though, is that you work consistently.

Keep a second point in mind: The line between extreme and routine doesn't hold still. Female athletes do things in gyms today that a previous generation of male athletes would've considered extreme. My rule of thumb: If you can do it without hurting or frustrating yourself, it's not too extreme. Don't judge or compare yourself against others. Extreme is where you and only you hit your limit. That's where I want you to hang out.

"He must be doing something compulsive. . . ." "Look at that guy. Anyone who looks like that has to be obsessed with his body. Exercise is okay, but there's no need to be compulsive about it."

I get that a lot, though never to my face. My guess is it's based on jealousy. People see something they think is beyond their reach, so they assign a pathology to it. Check out the logic: "That guy's so healthy that he must be sick."

Don't confuse determination and healthy habits with compulsion. You brush your teeth every day no matter what, and you probably feel uncomfortable when you can't do it for some reason. Does that mean you're obsessed with your teeth? Hell, no. It means you practice good dental hygiene.

In the chapters ahead, I'll urge you to make exercise a habit in your life, something you do almost automatically—like brushing your teeth. Turning exercise into a solid habit is the key to the Cover Model Workout or any other successful fitness program. Acquiring the habit calls for persistence and dedication. In the early stages, you'll have to force yourself to get your workout in on some days. But you'll do it.

If somebody interprets that as compulsive behavior, show him a dictionary. Then suggest that he stop throwing words like *compulsive* around so lightly.

"He must be doing something unhealthy, if not illegal. . . ." Let's not mince words. We know what they're talking about. They're saying I take steroids.

I don't. As God is my witness, I have never taken any performance-boosting or physique-enhancing supplement (not even creatine). And I never will use anything risky. I made a promise first to myself and then to my wife that I will never go that route. It's a promise that I won't break. If there's one thing I'm particularly proud of, it's being in the position I'm in without ever having used the juice. Not many guys can say that.

It's not that I'm applying for Boy Scout of the Year. It's just that steroids run contrary to all my deeply held convictions about physical health. The reason I won't touch them goes back to my original motivation for achieving maximum fitness: my dad's fatal heart attack at age 41. My goal was—and is—a long, healthy life. Steroids sabotage that goal. (Besides, they'd put more hair on my back, and God knows that's the last thing I need.)

I'm fully aware, though, that people are going to think I take steroids no matter what I say or do. That's part of the male-icon business. The steroid stigma is the most common of the nega-

"Extreme is where you and only you hit your limit. That's where I want you to hang out."

tive assumptions that haunt superfit guys. And you know what? I don't really blame people for thinking it. The truth is that guys in really phenomenal shape who aren't taking something are probably in the minority. 'Roids are so rampant that I and all the other guys who never touch the stuff are presumed guilty by association.

I mean, some of the most unhealthy people I've ever seen are competitive bodybuilders. Some of them are disciplined and work their butts off. I admire them for that. But they're so juiced up that I fear for their futures.

In my line of work, the competition for cover gigs is brutal, and plenty of guys won't hesitate to do whatever it takes to come out ahead. If that means dining at the East German café, they'll make their reservations early and often. So I not only go up against guys 10 or 15 years younger than I am but I have to overcome their synthetic testosterone advantage as well. I do all right, though, don't I? In fact, I'm living proof that you don't need performance-enhancing drugs to get yourself a head-turning, magazine-selling, awe-inspiring body. I've never done steroids and neither should you.

I've brought up all these stereotypes and misconceptions about male fitness for a couple of reasons. One is to set the record straight, which I hope I've done. The other is to clue you in on my recommended way to handle the inevitable naysayers. The temptation is to tell you to just ignore them. But you know what? It's better to do just the opposite: Inform them.

I listen to all the scrutinizers who look for

flaws in everything I do. Who knows? They may occasionally point out a true flaw that I can then try to correct. And if they're just jerking my chain, I can take that negativity and use it as motivation to work harder. Converting adversity to healthy motivation is part of my workout philosophy. It's something I'm going to urge you to do over and over again throughout this book. And you'll have a million occasions to put that philosophy into action as you follow my path to fitness.

Fitness from the Inside Out

I believe in achieving fitness from the inside out. That means developing your God-given physical capacity to its highest expression by providing your body with the nutrition it needs as you exercise it regularly and vigorously.

Inside-out training creates health, confidence, physical strength, and mental clarity. The benefits last a lifetime.

The opposite of inside-out training is the quick fix. Quick-fix seekers hope that something from the outside—a pill, a drug, a machine, a miracle diet—will deliver immediate results to their door, like a Federal Express truck. The benefits, if there are any, don't last.

Most people are looking for superficial results. They couldn't care less about health or strength or mental clarity. They just want to look better or lose weight or both. And they want it yesterday. I'm not knocking those people. But I am knocking the unscrupulous individuals who sell them that lie.

"Your body wants to be fit and strong and healthy. The power to get it that way is already there inside you, ready to go."

And believe me, it sells. That's why the media are saturated with ads for fad diets and gimmick machines and ab gizmos and all flavors of secret sauce. People want a quick fix so badly that they ignore how absurd it is for a product to claim to take inches off your waist in 24 hours. They're even willing to swallow the idea that an electronic stimulator can give you washboard abs.

You should be very wary of products that beat you over the head with before-and-after pictures. None of that stuff is worth 2 seconds of your time. Trust me on this. The quick-fix approach will leave you worse off than when you started. Even if you do manage to lose weight fast on some kind of flash diet, you're always going to gain it back—but only after you've subjected your body to unnecessary abuse.

You know what's the most insidious thing about all this? The quick fixes that "work" are the worst of all. Steroids and speedy drugs and some other supplements, legal and illegal, will help you simulate the outward appearance of a lean and muscled human being. But it's not the look of a healthy man. It's the look of a man with chemically induced heart palpitations, a man with haywire metabolism, a man in hormone hell. A man heading for early death.

When you train my way—from the inside out—you steer clear of those pitfalls by focusing on your entire being instead of your appearance. The benefits of working from the inside out go way beyond aesthetics. They reach your soul. You're not in this just for looks.

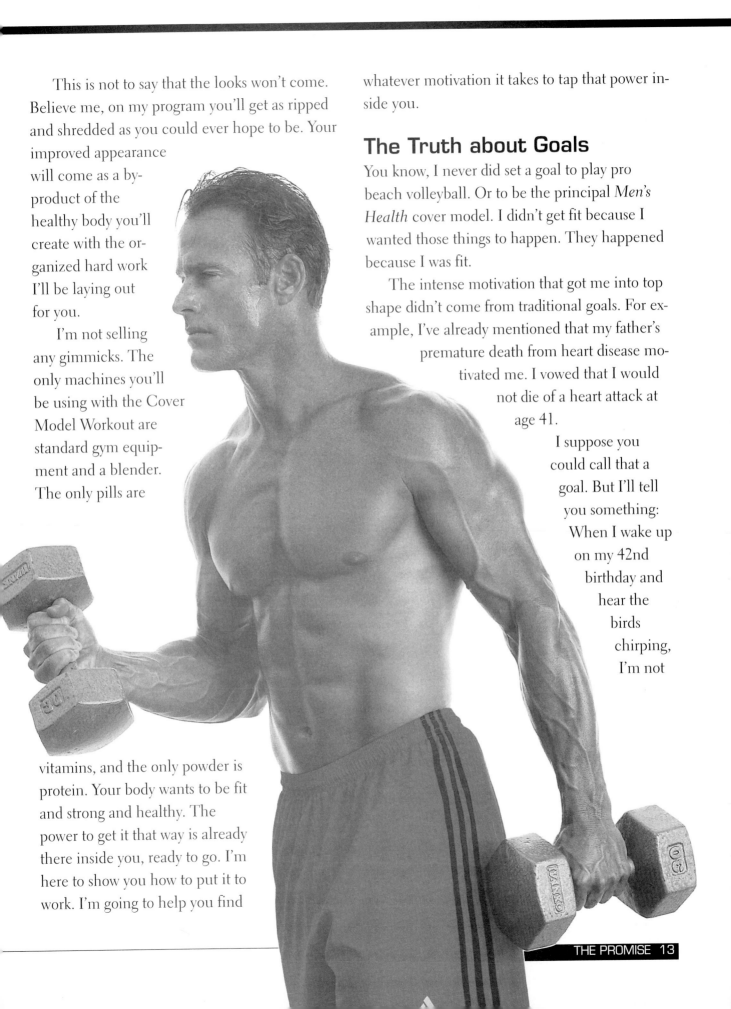

This is not to say that the looks won't come. Believe me, on my program you'll get as ripped and shredded as you could ever hope to be. Your improved appearance will come as a by-product of the healthy body you'll create with the organized hard work I'll be laying out for you.

I'm not selling any gimmicks. The only machines you'll be using with the Cover Model Workout are standard gym equipment and a blender. The only pills are vitamins, and the only powder is protein. Your body wants to be fit and strong and healthy. The power to get it that way is already there inside you, ready to go. I'm here to show you how to put it to work. I'm going to help you find whatever motivation it takes to tap that power inside you.

The Truth about Goals

You know, I never did set a goal to play pro beach volleyball. Or to be the principal *Men's Health* cover model. I didn't get fit because I wanted those things to happen. They happened because I was fit.

The intense motivation that got me into top shape didn't come from traditional goals. For example, I've already mentioned that my father's premature death from heart disease motivated me. I vowed that I would not die of a heart attack at age 41.

I suppose you could call that a goal. But I'll tell you something: When I wake up on my 42nd birthday and hear the birds chirping, I'm not going to kick back because I've reached a goal. That will happen only when I die in bed of natural causes at age 102 with my family around me.

What I'm getting at is this: Maximum fitness—and the health that goes with it—is its own reward. In my opinion, the only worthwhile goal of a fitness program is to be as fit and healthy as you can be. I don't outright condemn the more concrete goals. If getting down to your high school

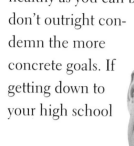

waist size before the upcoming reunion motivates you to start the Cover Model Workout and then stick with it—hey, go for it. Whatever it takes.

I have goals like that whenever I'm scheduled for a cover shoot. Time is usually tight, and there's often a certain look I need to achieve. It becomes a short-term, concrete goal that influences my workout and diet. So I'd be the last guy to trivialize that kind of goal.

But I do say be careful. Some goals can eclipse your fitness quest if you let them. If getting into those smaller pants is all that matters to you, you might be tempted to get there in ways that do your health no good—a crash diet or water depletion or sacrificing muscle mass along with the fat.

Goals can also have an even more harmful effect. They can set you up for failure if they're not based on what a fitness program actually accomplishes. No fitness program can get you a whole new body that conforms to some predetermined notion of what you want it to look like. Instead, exercise improves the body you have. That body will respond magnificently if you challenge it regularly. But it will always respond in its own way and within its own limitations.

What's more, you can't tell in advance just what that response will be, what your body will look like when it's in the best shape possible. Maybe after a few months of workouts you'll look almost the same as when you started—but with a dramatic increase in strength. Maybe you'll respond more to the cardiovascular exercises than to the weight training and, in the process, discover a passion for endurance exercise that goes with your new, leaner body. Maybe your newfound fitness will help you in your career. Or maybe you'll find that your current career isn't compatible with exercise.

Exercise will help you discover something about yourself that you can't foresee. All you'll know is that you'll feel better and be healthier when you get there.

You want real goals? Helpful goals? I'll give you fitness goals that will do some good. Today, instead of a goal to reach a certain waist size or look like a cover model, your goal is to get to the gym and work out as hard as you can. Tomorrow, your goal will be the same. Instead of obsessing about long-term goals, focus on the rewards of actually doing your daily workout. Let your goal be to complete what you need to do in the gym that day. The purpose of a goal is to motivate you. Using a goal to replace motivation is the quickest way to failure.

"Exercise will help you discover something about yourself that you can't foresee."

The Icon Will See You Now

I do a lot of motivating. I'm good at it.

When I'm at a party or soaking in a hot tub somewhere, and I start talking with somebody who has some problems, before long he's getting the full spiel. I tell him what to do and what not to do, what to eat and what not to eat. By the time I'm through with him, the guy is a raging brushfire of enthusiasm.

Then I run into him a few months later and the results are astonishing. The guy looks 10 years younger. He's bursting with confidence. He's a new man. I can't begin to tell you what a rush that is. It's gratifying that people even listen to me in the first place. But when I'm able to get guys motivated enough to implement my advice and rediscover their sense of self-worth, I get off on that a lot more than seeing myself on a cover. That, to me, is the best part of being in the position I'm in.

I've written this book to give you the same motivation and confidence. My plan is pretty simple: I'm going to explain to you what the Cover Model Workout is all about and why it will work for you. I'm going to tell you about the bizarre trajectory of my life that fueled my motivation and led to the creation of the Cover Model Workout. I'm going to show you what I did to get myself into cover model shape. Finally, I'm going to take you through the best version of the Cover Model Workout for you and your body.

What I'm *not* going to do is turn you into an Owen McKibbin clone. Even if such a thing were possible, you wouldn't want it. I'm offering all the tools you need to become a stronger, healthier, fitter, more self-confident you. But it will still be *you*—100 percent, genuine, unadulterated you. Maybe there really is a cover model inside you waiting to emerge. More likely, there's a leaner, harder, more athletic-looking version of what you look like now. Whatever it is, I guarantee you'll like it more than what you see now.

Welcome to the Cover Model Workout

When I use the phrase *Cover Model Workout*, I'm talking about a complete physical-fitness program for you to follow step by step. The program progresses steadily over a period of at least 4 months, so you'll continue to see improvement as you keep meeting new challenges. After you work your way through the entire program, not only will you be in the best shape of your life but you'll have mastered the tools and workout structure to maintain your peak fitness level for the rest of your life.

As I reveal my workout methods in the chapters ahead, I'll share with you the details and secrets of the training methods that I've developed over 20 years. These strategies have worked for me in good times and bad. They'll work for you, too, whether you're a raw beginner or a grizzled veteran.

In return, I'm asking two things of you.

1. I want you to give me 3 to 5 hours of your time each week. You can spread those hours over 3 days or 6 days, but you must be absolutely consistent about alloting that amount of time to your workouts.

    In truth, you won't "give me" those hours. You'll dedicate them to your health, your appearance, and your overall well-being.

2. I want you to pay attention to what you feed your body. Promise me that your first priority will be to eat food that will help you achieve your fitness goals, and avoid food that will sabotage those goals.

When you make those two simple commitments, you're ready to dive headfirst into my program and take it for all it's worth. For all the fine-tuning I've done over the years, the basic structure of my program is simple. Here's what you'll do for the rest of your life.

→ You'll burn off body fat, extend your endurance, and toughen your tendons and ligaments with cardiovascular exercise at least 3 days a week. Sometimes called aerobic exercise, cardio can be walking,

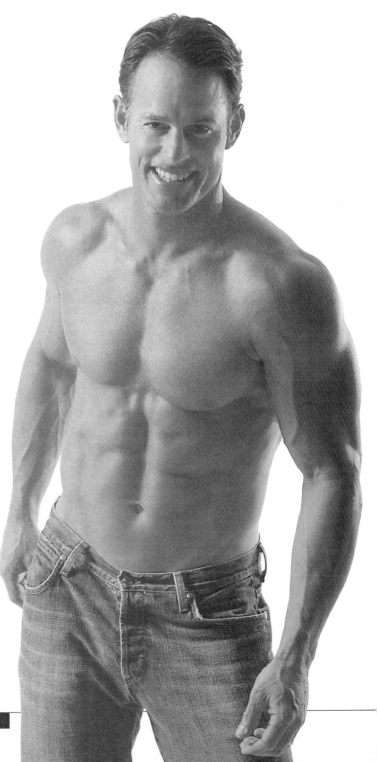

jogging, cycling, swimming laps—anything that gets your heart and lungs pumping. I'll mix up your cardio sessions: Sometimes I'll have you go at a steady pace for 40 minutes, other times you'll do quick sprints on and off for about 20 minutes.

→ You'll build lean muscle proportionately throughout your body via three 30- to 45-minute weight-training sessions per week. Two of those sessions will focus on developing the "core" muscles that show: your upper back, chest, arms, and legs. The third session (what I call the integrity workout) will get at the smaller muscles around your joints and elsewhere that are vital to moving fluidly and avoiding injury. All three strength-training sessions will get rid of flab as they build muscle, because all that new lean body mass will jack up your metabolism so you burn calories more efficiently.

→ You'll solidify your lean look and tap into energy reserves you never knew you had

"I'll share with you the details and secrets of the training methods that I've developed over 20 years."

by following the nutrition guidelines I'll give you. I'm not peddling any gimmick diets or calorie-deprivation regimens. I will show you how to gradually reduce your intake of the foods that do the most harm, especially the high-glycemic carbohydrates such as bread, pasta, potatoes, and rice. And I'll provide you with ways to eat more of the foods that will actually help you build muscle and shed fat.

Those are the basics of your Cover Model Workout: cardio work 3 days a week, weight training 3 days a week, and smart eating 6 days a week (with permission to treat yourself to a diet "cheat day" once a week). Is it really that simple? You bet.

By the time you finish reading this book, you'll know more about the best methods for getting into peak condition than 99.9 percent of the people on this planet. More important, you'll be practicing those methods.

So let's get started.

THE PRINCIPLES

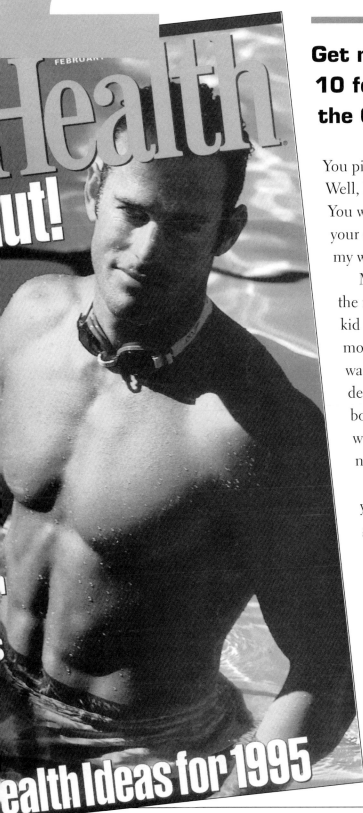

FEBRUARY

Health

ut!

ealth Ideas for 1995

**Get ready to learn the
10 founding principles of
the Cover Model Workout.**

You picked up this book to get a better body, right? Well, I'm going to show you exactly how to do that. You won't end up with *my* body. You'll end up with your own best body, but you're going to get there my way.

My Cover Model Workout has been 20 years in the making. I didn't get from there (a nearly crippled kid facing years of hard-core pain) to here (the very model of health and fitness) because my regimen was state-of-the-art from the beginning. It took 2 decades of trial and error, close observation, a bit of borrowing, and a train wreck of a life for my workout to evolve to what I'll be presenting in the next part of this book.

But for all the fine-tuning I've done over the years, the bedrock principles of my fitness program have never changed. Why should they? They've kept me in cover model condition through all the ups and downs of my never-dull existence. They've shaped up everybody I've ever trained. And when you get into the program, they'll reward your hard efforts with a leaner, muscled body and a newfound energy that will seem unlimited.

I'll run through these principles for you here because, taken as a whole, they're what distinguish my fitness program from all the rest. Then I'll explain how they fit into the workouts you'll be doing. Basically, they come down to 10 things I firmly believe about health and fitness.

1. I believe that cardiovascular exercise and strength training are equally important for everybody—no matter which you prefer, no matter which is trendier at the moment, and no matter what type of body you have.

2. I believe in diet as an essential component of fitness, not merely a support strategy.

3. I believe that exercise done in hard, short bursts will get you into better shape, and get you there faster, than long, slow efforts.

4. I believe that weight-lifting sessions targeting the big muscles must be interspersed with workouts that focus on strengthening the smaller, more injury-prone muscles and joints.

5. I believe that muscles should be developed for function, not just display.

6. I believe that an overemphasis on crunches and situps is not the way to work your midsection and achieve washboard abs.

7. I believe in drinking buckets of water all day long.

8. I believe in stretching as a fitness necessity, not as a warmup, cooldown, or ancillary activity.

9. I believe in rest but not necessarily in rest days.

10. I believe in clean living.

Now let's take a closer look at each of these components. Get to know them. They're going to be part of your life from now on.

1. Cardio and Strength Training Are Equally Important

Most guys lean toward one of these two training modes more than the other, and I'm no exception. When you're carrying around a gene that predisposes you to early death from cardiac disease, you're going to favor the form of exercise that strengthens the most important muscle in your body: your heart. That's what cardiovascular exercise does.

When I talk about cardio, I mean the kind of endurance exercise that raises your heart rate for a sustained period of time as you use oxygen to burn fat for energy. That can be walking, running, cycling, stairclimbing, cross-country skiing, aerobic dancing, and a bunch of other things. It can also be the machine equivalent of those activities, like stationary bikes or treadmills.

It doesn't matter which you do, but it does matter that you do it regularly. You can get washboard abs without ever doing one situp, but you absolutely cannot get washboard abs without consistent cardio work. A lot of guys like weight training best, and that's fine. But you have to do your cardio too. Without it, there's no Cover Model Workout.

Cardio is especially important for beginners because it thickens the tendons and ligaments in your joints to get you ready for higher-intensity, more ballistic exercise. It also helps you shed flab, increases your capacity to use oxygen, and improves your endurance. Need I add that you'll be doing a lot of cardio in this program?

But as gung-ho as I am about cardio, I know I'd be cheating myself if I didn't focus just as heavily on strength training—which is sometimes called resistance training but mostly referred to as lifting weights. It's the fitness component that builds your muscle mass and strength. I'm figuring I don't need to convince you why that's a big part of the workout.

But you should know that resistance training does a lot more than bulge your muscles. It strengthens your bones, pumps up your natural testosterone release, sharpens your central nervous system, and improves your cardiovascular health by building stronger limbs that make life easier on your heart. And resistance training gets more important—not less—as you get older. You lose muscle mass and bone density with the years. Lifting weights offsets those losses.

Clearly, cardio and strength training are both key to the kind of fitness you're trying to achieve. So why do I feel the need to emphasize their equal importance? For some guys, getting lean is their top fitness priority. They know that cardio work and eating right are the keys to shedding body fat. So a lot of them conclude that resistance training doesn't fit into their plans. Some even mistakenly believe that building muscle will work against them, as though muscle and body fat were the same thing.

But added muscle actually helps fight flab because it jacks up your metabolism so you burn more calories throughout the day. Just as important, losing fat is a tainted victory if that's all you do. Let's face it, being thin and weak isn't really

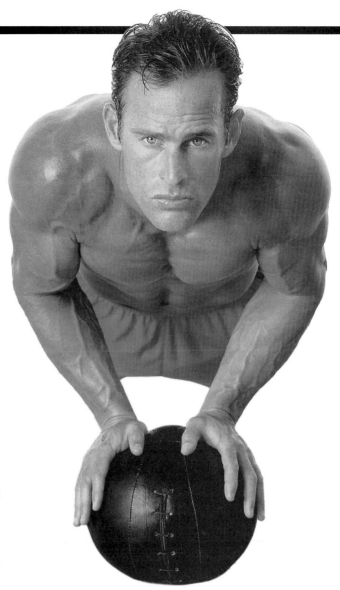

being in shape. You're still not healthy. You have to build muscle.

Then there's the group on the other side of the fence, the "ironheads" who consider 20 minutes on a stationary bike to be 20 minutes wasted. Gyms usually have on view living examples of the pitfalls of overemphasizing weight training at the expense of cardio work. You see pot-bellied guys who lift like lunatics but have never walked farther than the distance from one weight stack to the next. These guys have muscles the size of college dorm rooms, but they're as far from a *Men's Health* cover as those lonely long-distance runners—probably even farther. And the marathoners will probably live longer. Nobody has ever died from skinny arms. But an undertrained heart muscle combined with obesity will put you under quick.

Guys who do nothing but lift tend to get soft in the middle. They often don't care about being lean, so they're not. And they're not as healthy as they should be. But even the ones who aren't soft and flabby—like most serious bodybuilders—are still missing something. They don't look right, in my book, especially the really big ones.

I have to emphasize that these are extreme examples I'm describing. There's nothing wrong at all with preferring weight training over cardio work. For some guys, lifting a weight is a more satisfying effort than sprinting up hills or pounding a treadmill. This becomes a problem only if they start neglecting their cardio training for more muscle work.

The program in this book will help you avoid that trap. You need the right balance between strength training and cardio work, and my workout is based on that balance.

I don't think there's any substitute for the body in motion. For me, moving a dumbbell a few feet is an excellent strength-training exercise—but it doesn't come close to expressing the human capacity for movement.

If you put a gun to my head and made me choose between lifting and sprinting, I'd head straight for The Hill and never see a weight room again. The natural movements that go with most modes of cardio work reflect themselves in a certain elegance of gait that pure weight lifters don't have. If all you do is lift weights, you're going to walk in a way that makes people say, "Weight lifter!" That's not the same as saying, "That guy's in great shape!"

Let me put it another way. Watch a cat sometimes—a black panther at the zoo or your neighbor's housecat. What do you see? You see a well-muscled, smooth-moving, rhythmically gaited animal. That, to me, is the essence of a well-balanced weight and cardio regimen. The gait you'll develop from blending weight and cardio work in the Cover Model Workout is your badge of honor. You'll walk with your shoulders back, chest out, stomach in tight, and head held high—as though a cape were flowing off your back. It's not a strut or a swagger. It's 100 percent natural. Your walk tells the world that you can handle anything it throws at you. You're confident and proud of who you are.

"You need the right balance between strength training and cardio work, and my workout is based on that balance."

2. The Power of Eating Right

Eating right isn't something you do to support your fitness program. It's *part* of your fitness program. Diet is as essential a component of the Cover Model Workout as cardio exercise and strength training. Simply put, if you don't eat right, you won't get fit.

By no means am I talking about a calorie-deprivation diet where you keep yourself hungry all the time so that you'll lose weight. That's a recipe for disaster. I'm talking about eating good foods in the right amounts at the best times.

The idea is to fuel your workouts, give your muscles the food they need to grow, and find a balance where you burn at least as many calories as you take in—which is the only way to get rid of the flab around your midsection.

The eating plan I'll outline in part three is loaded with food options. So don't worry; I'm going to feed you well. I'm also going to urge you to pay attention to *when* you eat. I take an early dinner and make sure I don't eat high-glycemic carbohydrates (such as pasta or bread) after the sun goes down. Those carbs convert quickly to sugar that your body will store as fat if you don't work it off. If I eat high-glycemic carbs at night, I wake up feeling bloated. But give me a lean steak and vegetables without the potato for dinner, and I swear I wake up leaner, with a flatter stomach, than when I went to bed.

3. Short and Hard Beats Long and Slow

Lifting weights is by its very nature an activity of short, hard efforts. But in my workouts, you're going to get to the point where even your cardio work will stress the advantages of the short-burst approach. Why? Because it will get you in shape faster. And it will pay off in your upper-body development. I'm a big admirer of marathoners, and I know I could never do what they do. But

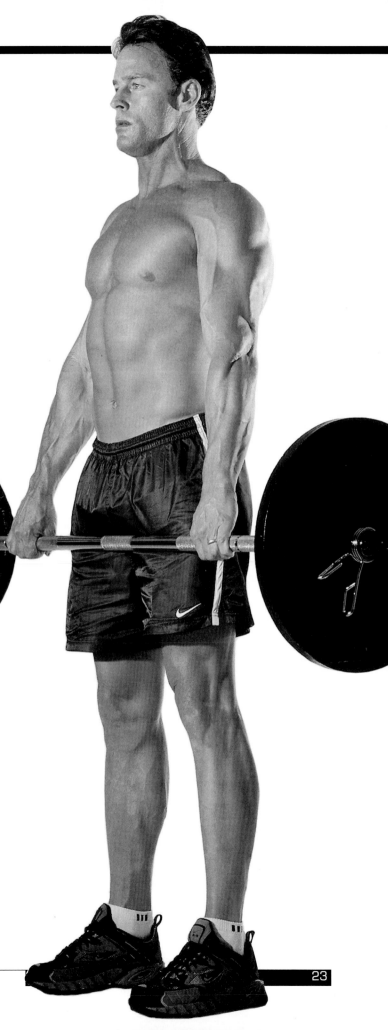

I'd be out of a job if I looked like those guys. There's just not much of a market for skinny models with sunken chests. It's way too late for me to do the waif thing you see in so many ads. Besides, I get bored doing traditional cardio work such as running long distances or pedaling an exercise bike at a steady pace for 45 minutes. At the same time, I want to burn fat and reap all the other benefits of aerobic exercise.

My solution is sprinting. Sprinting is the quintessential Cover Model Workout exercise. By definition, it's a short-burst effort. If you can do sprints one after another for much more than 20 minutes, you're not sprinting hard enough. By sprinting, I mean an all-out, hard-as-you-can-go, straight-ahead effort for 10 to 30 seconds, followed by a slowdown or short rest, and then another sprint while your heart rate is still high enough for the fat-burning aerobic effect to continue. You can do sprints on a bicycle or in the pool, but I encourage you to do running sprints—preferably on grass, sand, or some kind of running track to spare your joints the pounding from pavement. You use more of your body when actually running your sprints, and your mind is better focused on the action.

If you don't believe me, take a look at a sprinter's body. A lot of sprinters could blow me off the cover. Then check them out in action. Their arms are churning, their knees are pumping like pistons, their trunks are rotating. They're blasting their abs, their hamstrings, their quads, and their calves. All muscles are firing and working together.

4. The Hidden Muscles Need Work as Much as the Big Guys

The kind of injury that will put you out of commission isn't likely to be a problem with your big muscle groups, like the lats and traps on your back or the pectorals across your chest. When guys go down, it's almost always because they've injured rotator cuff muscles, or something in their lower backs, or ligaments or tendons around their knee or elbow joints. A big reason that happens is because they never bother training the little

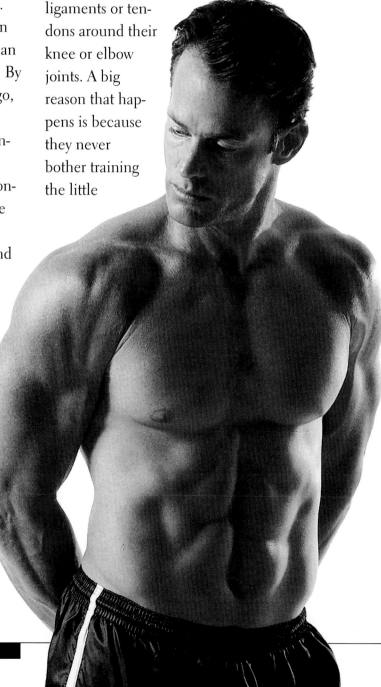

muscles that protect those areas. You will.

Not to criticize, but Mother Nature didn't do a perfect job in constructing our elbows, knees, and shoulders, and the risk of injury increases with the volume and intensity of exercise. That's why my workout stresses the importance of strengthening the joint-area muscles you don't see, as well as the big-money muscles. I've found it works best to separate your lifting efforts into "integrity" days, when you emphasize the small muscles, and "core" days, when you do your heavy lifting. This will give you an advantage over the guys who take their joints and little muscles for granted until they're hurt.

5. Build Muscles You Can Use

I make my living by looking good, but that's not the only reason I bust my butt in the weight room. I want my muscles to be useful, not just big. What's the point of putting in all that time with inert slabs of iron if you can't push guys out of the paint or hit your receiver downfield?

I'm not saying your priority should be the same. I don't care why you lift weights, as long as you do it consistently. Still, the resistance programs in the Cover Model Workout emphasize muscle performance over sheer muscle size. That's why you'll do most of the lifts with free weights instead of machines. And that's why you'll do more compound movements than isolation lifts that focus on one muscle group only.

A perfect example of the kind of compound move I'm talking about is the pullup, a movement so natural you don't even use a weight. Here your upper-back and biceps muscles work together to move your body against gravity. It's a move you can use. I believe religiously in

pullups. They're the most satisfying upper-body exercise there is. They're also the most strenuous. You don't see lines at the pullup bar in any gym I've entered.

6. Awesome Abs without (Too Many) Situps and Crunches

I see way too many guys wasting their time doing hundreds of crunches every day because they think that's the route to a flat, hard stomach. It's not. They'd be better off using most of that time to work the rest of their body musculature and to do their cardio. Reducing your body-fat percentage is the secret to washboard abs. Diet, cardio, and metabolism-boosting strength exercises—not situps—get the job done. You can get your bitchin' six-pack without ever doing a situp.

If you want to know the truth, too many crunches or situps can be counterproductive. That goes for the twist or sideways versions that work the oblique muscles of your sides. You might end up building up your stomach area and getting a thick-in-the-middle look you don't want.

Trust me, I had to learn this the hard way. Check out the November 2000 *Men's Health* cover. I was doing far too much oblique work—doing so many side crunches and twists that I had actually built my obliques to the point that I looked like I had love handles. That's when I came around to the idea that you should work your abs and obliques the way you sear a good piece of tuna on a grill. Boom-boom, a minute or two on each side, and that's it. I cut back on the ab work, and it tapered my waistline and made my shoulders appear wider.

7. Tons of Water Will Work Wonders

I am a major advocate of drinking as much water as you can throughout the day. I'm convinced that one of the reasons for my success over the years is all the water I pour down my throat. To follow the Cover Model Workout, you must drink a lot of water.

Water moves food through your system so you don't feel bloated. It rehydrates your cells so your eyes aren't dry, your skin feels good, and your throat doesn't bother you. It regulates your body temperature.

All those are terrific benefits, but the biggest one may be that the more water you drink, the less water your body holds beneath your skin. Here's a weird example: Ever notice how your wife/girlfriend/coworker complains that she gets "fat" at a certain time of the month. It's not that she's suddenly put on a few pounds of adipose tissue. Her body is simply holding water in anticipation of her period.

Guys don't have periods (let's count our blessings), but we do tend to hold water beneath our skin, particularly after eating salty foods. If you notice your weight fluctuating from one day to the next, or if you see that some days you look puffier than usual, that's your body holding water. And, paradoxical as it sounds, you need water to lose water.

Give water a chance next time you think about chugging a soda. Squeeze a little lemon in it, drink it down, and see if you still need that Coke. Same thing next time you're going out for beers. Quench your thirst first with a great big glass of water. You'll enjoy the beer more even as you drink less.

You've probably heard that you need six to eight glasses of water a day to stay healthy. The way I see it, if you can count the glasses, you aren't drinking enough. I down about 2 gallons of water a day. Fair warning: Getting stuck in traffic can really be a problem. So when you know you have to spend a couple of hours without a urinal in sight, you have my permission to shut off the spigot. Other than those times, though, I want you to drink water all day long—before, during, and after meals, and especially during and after your workouts.

8. Stretching Pays Off Big Time

First—and obviously—a consistent stretching program will work wonders for your flexibility. That pays off all day long, every day, as it makes all of life's typical motions—reaching, twisting, crouching, craning, thrusting, and so on—so much easier. It also pays off in the gym, where the increased range of motion translates into more productive lifts.

Personally, I believe stretching protects your joints; soothes tight, irritated muscles; and often prevents post-workout soreness. These aren't proven benefits—it's hard to prove anything when it comes to flexibility, since it's such a situational, technique-driven form of exercise—but that's how it works with my body, using my stretching routine.

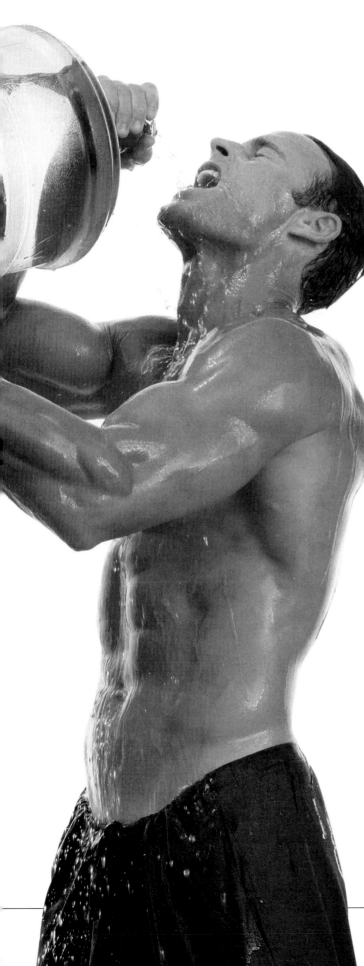

I do four different types of stretches, in four different situations. First is ballistic stretching—like those big arm circles or head-and-neck rotations that you see swimmers do before jumping into the pool—which I do as part of my warmup for a swim or weight-lifting workout.

The idea here is to get my muscles and joints lubed up and ready to work in a full range of motion.

The second type is static stretching, in which I go into the deep stretches shown on pages 28 to 30 and hold those positions for up to a minute. I do these after my workouts, when my muscles and joints are as warm and supple as they'll ever be. I think this type of stretching not only improves my overall flexibility but also prevents excessive stiffness and soreness. I can tell the difference when I don't stretch after a workout.

The lower-body stretches are a key part of my program. Make sure you hit the hamstrings on the backs of your thighs, the quadriceps on the fronts, your calves, your groin, your glutes, and your lower back. Upper-body stretches combine your shoulders with your triceps and your chest.

Third, I stretch my muscles in between sets at the gym. For example, after sets of pullups, I like to hang from the bar to stretch out my shoulders and lats.

Finally, I do stretches all day long, just about wherever I am. I stretch my shoulders as the hot water beats down on them in the shower. I stretch in the steam room. I stop and do calf stretches just about anywhere. These aren't aggressive stretches designed for any type of performance benefit. They just feel good.

The Stretches

HAMSTRING AND LOWER-BACK STRETCH

Sit on the floor with one leg straight out in front of you. Hook a towel around the ball of that foot and hold the ends. Bend your other knee and place the sole of that foot against the side of your extended leg. Gently yet firmly pull on the towel ends to stretch your upper body toward your extended foot. Hold for 1 minute, then repeat with the opposite leg extended.

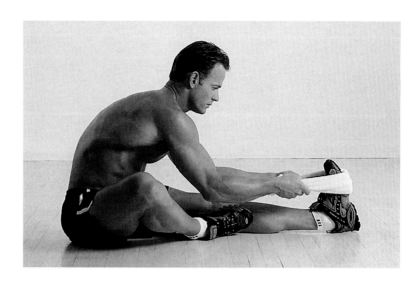

QUADRICEPS STRETCH

Stand up straight, bend one knee, and reach behind you to grab the instep of your raised foot. Keeping your knees parallel to each other, pull your heel toward your butt. Hold for 1 minute, then repeat with your other foot raised.

CALVES, ACHILLES, AND HAMSTRINGS STRETCH

From a standing position, bend down and place your palms flat on the floor. Slowly walk your feet back until you feel a deep stretch along the entire back side of your lower body. To stretch your Achilles tendons farther, slowly bend one knee and then the other, allowing your heels to lift off the floor. Hold for 1 minute.

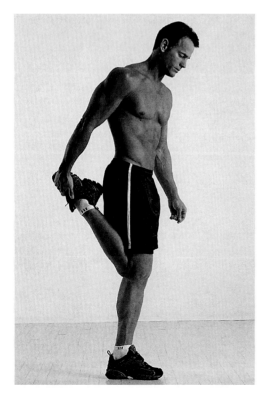

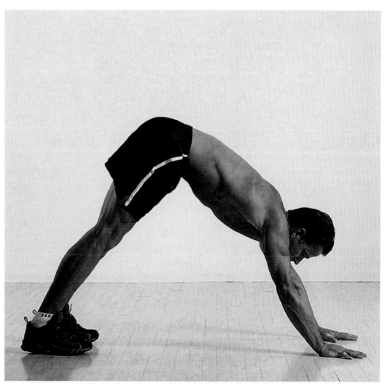

GROIN STRETCH

Sit on the floor and press together the soles of your feet, with your knees bent and pointing out to the sides. Keeping your back as straight as possible, place your hands on your upper ankles and slowly press your elbows down on the insides of your thighs. Don't bounce. Hold for 1 minute.

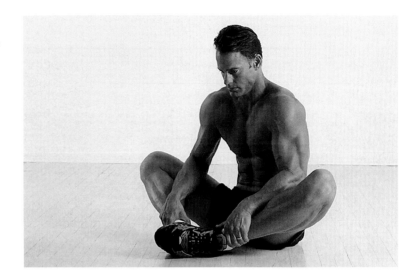

GLUTES STRETCH

Lie on the floor with one knee bent and that foot flat on the floor. Place the ankle of your other foot against your bent knee. Slowly bring your bent knee toward your head. Hold for 1 minute, then repeat on your other side.

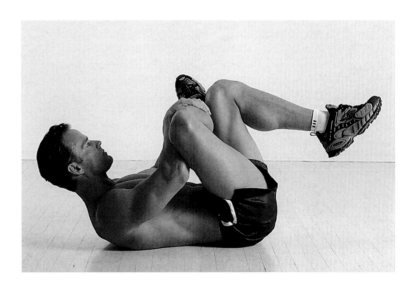

LOWER-BACK STRETCH

Lie flat on the floor with your arms stretched up above your head. Slowly raise your knees to your chest. Extend your feet up over your head, letting them fall behind your head and trying to touch your toes to the floor. Gradually increase the distance between your feet and head. Hold for 1 minute.

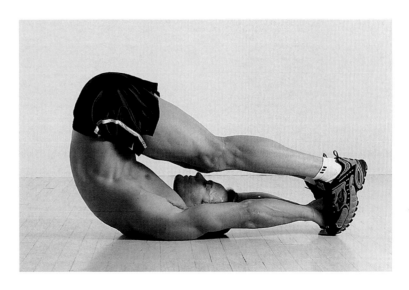

SHOULDER STRETCH

Stand up straight and cross one arm across your chest. Use your other arm to apply pressure to just above the elbow of your crossed arm. Hold for 1 minute, then switch arms.

SHOULDERS-AND-TRICEPS STRETCH

Stand up straight and lift one arm so your elbow is bent next to your ear. Lower your hand as far down your back as possible. Use your other hand to apply pressure just above the elbow of your reaching arm. Hold for 1 minute, then switch arms.

CHEST-AND-SHOULDER STRETCH

Stand up straight and clasp your hands behind your butt. Pull your shoulder blades together and push your chest outward. Hold for 1 minute.

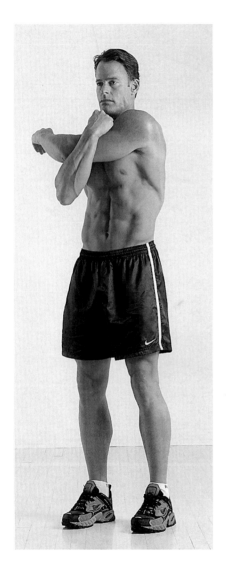

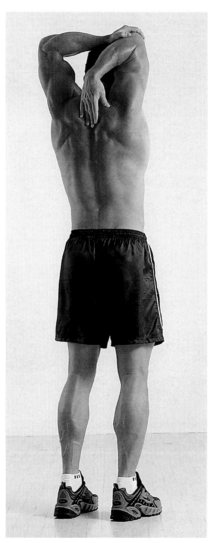

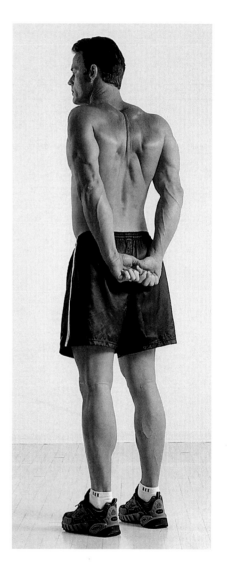

9. Get the Most out of Your Rest

Rest is a lot more important than you may think. Resistance training works because your muscles respond to the stress you put on them by making themselves bigger and stronger than they were before. That growth happens only during rest. And that's why it's foolish to work the same muscle groups 2 days in a row. The Cover Model Workout gives you plenty of rest between workouts.

Sleep, too, is key. As your healthy eating and hard exercise become a regimen, you'll sleep like a baby. You'll fall asleep earlier and wake up earlier, and your body will repair itself better in between. That deep rest then helps you work out even harder the next day. It's a win-win cycle. For all my extreme ways, I'm as kicked-back as a guy can be once the workouts are in and the day is done—you practically have to check me for a pulse. I appreciate rest. But I have to admit, my idea of rest doesn't include a complete day off. I just don't feel right if I don't do some kind of exercise every day. I'm always going to find a way to steal some.

With the Cover Model Workout, you can go ahead and take a rest day once a week—even twice if you double up the resistance and cardio workouts. But again, don't blow off everything on those days of "rest." Eat right. Drink tons of water. Do some stretches.

10. Clean Living Is an Ally

To me, clean living means respect for your body. It means respect for yourself. And it means re-

spect for others. What does it have to do with a fitness program? Everything. For a long time, I separated my lifestyle from my fitness pursuits—and, yes, I got away with it . . . for a while. But as you'll see in the next chapter, it really wasn't until I woke up from major back surgery with a rock-solid desire to clean up my act that I was able to attain the truly vibrant fitness that put me on the cover of *Men's Health* and in front of the television cameras.

I urge you to make the same commitment to clean living that I did. I consider it an essential component of the Cover Model Workout. If your muscles are your body's engine, clean living is your carburetor. Clean eating gives you the best fuel for your muscles. A clean social life (notice I didn't say "nonexistent" social life) allows you to have fun but still get plenty of sleep and wake up refreshed and ready for the day.

When you live clean, you not only have better workouts but also get more benefits from workouts: more energy, more focus, more life. I'll show in the next chapter what a party dog I used to be. And in the chapter after that I'll show how—and why—I cleaned up my act. For now, let me just say this much: I'm having a much better time now than I ever did when I was trying to have so much fun. The better I treat my body, the more I enjoy life. Clean living is more fun than the alternative.

That said, I'll add that I have a couple of beers with buddies, a glass of wine with my wife at dinner, or a piece of cake at a birthday party. When I do, I enjoy them just as much as any-

> *"As your healthy eating and hard exercise become a regimen, you'll sleep like a baby."*

body does—maybe more, since they're treats for me, rather than part of my everyday life. Clean living isn't deprivation; it's choosing the right time and place for your indulgences.

The Mental Side of Physical Fitness

That's the physical part of the Cover Model Workout. To be honest, you can get workout and lifestyle tips anywhere, from anyone. I prefer mine to the alternatives, but you can still get great results from lots of different programs—if you follow them consistently.

Big "if," right? We'd all be ripped and rock hard if it were as easy as picking up a piece of paper, taking it to the gym, following the workout on the paper, and then repeating. Most people quit long before they get any results. About 50 percent of people quit an exercise program within the first 6 months, and about 75 percent give up within a year. Here is where I think I can help you the most. The nuts and bolts of the Cover Model Workout evolved along with my attitude about exercise and fitness. The mental and physical aspects of the program are inseparable. That's why understanding and implementing my mental approach to physical fitness is key to your success. If you get into it with the same mindset that I do, you're going to nail this workout and get every possible benefit from it.

If you don't approach it my way—if, instead, you treat it as just another set of workouts from just another buff guy—you'll still get something out of it. And anything is better than nothing. But everything is a lot better than either one.

I ask you to think of this workout as a beautiful, powerful animal that you have to approach with the right attitude and expectations. I've spent my life getting to know what's involved in carrying out a fitness program, and I've narrowed it down to the following five steps.

Step 1: Tap your motivation. If you're truly motivated to get yourself into top shape, you'll sail though my program. If you lack motivation, you'll tend to struggle. My hunch is that you're plenty motivated. You picked up this book, didn't you? What I don't know is the source of your motivation. But you should. And whatever led you to embark on this journey of health and fitness is something you can tap into to keep yourself working hard, on good days and bad. Constantly remind yourself why you're getting up early to do cardio, why you're drastically reducing bread and pasta in your diet, why you're pushing weights instead of the buttons on your TV's remote control. If you can't express your motivation in one sentence, take a little time for some introspection. Ask yourself what it is that has prompted you to take up the Cover Model Workout. Be honest with yourself. Are you in this to improve your health? Your appearance? Do you want to show up a rival or impress a woman? Are you aiming to bump me off the cover of *Men's Health*? Whatever it is—positive or negative, realistic or otherwise—keep reminding yourself why you're in this thing. Milk your motivation for all it's worth.

My way: Enlist the fear factor. My original motivation to get in perfect shape was fear. I feared an early death, like my father's. I feared the heart disease gene in my family and vowed to defeat it. Later, I feared obesity as I saw it developing in my older siblings. I even feared having skinny legs. Alternately gloomy and goofy stuff, I admit. But like I said, any motivation works as long as it results in a positive outcome. And there's no denying that my fears got the job done.

I've tapped into other sources of motivation as well. One is a fierce competitive streak, which probably started with my older brothers roughing me up all the time. I was motivated to get into the best shape possible because I wanted to win—against my brothers at first, then in soccer, then in volleyball, and now in full-court basketball and other pickup games.

Also, of course, there were the *Men's Health* covers. There's no better motivation for getting into shape than having your livelihood depend on it.

Step 2: Force yourself to get in the habit. If you're starting out, the first thing you have to do is acquire the habit of eating right and exercising just about every day. That's hard at first, like any new habit. But it's absolutely necessary. And you can do it. There's no getting around it: For the first month or so, you're going to have to force yourself to get it done. Think back to when you were a kid and your mom was all over you to brush your teeth every night. You hated it, but she made you do it. And then what happened? It became a habit, something you do now without thinking about it.

That's what has to happen with your fitness program, although now you have to do it without your mom nagging you.

You need to acquire this habit by any means possible. If you have the means and inclination to hire a personal trainer to ride your butt, go for

it. If you have to exercise less than I recommend in this program, that's what you have to do. It may take you months to work up to the amount of exercise required for the first phase of the Cover Model Workout. But if that's the best you can do, then you must do it. You can establish the habit with just a few minutes of exercise a day, as long as the exercise is done consistently and purposefully, with the goal of increasing volume and intensity.

I'm flexible on the type and volume of exercise you do at first—you have to trust your own instincts and respect your abilities. I think the workouts in this book will be appropriate for most guys, but for some, I'll concede, they're too much to start with. (And for a few, they may not be enough.)

But on one point I'm completely rigid. I'm a dictator for consistent, habitual exercise. If the best you can do is a 10-minute walk 5 days a week, with a half-dozen pushups and 10 crunches Monday, Wednesday, and Friday, that's what I expect you to do. Within a month, you should be up to a 15-minute walk, 10 pushups, and two dozen crunches. And within another month, you should be ready for the workout as I've designed it.

I don't care how hard it is to achieve this habit. And I won't sugarcoat it for you: Some days it's going to be brutal. It's 5 o'clock, you're flipping the channels, you're tired, dinner's cooking. You're happy where you are. Doesn't matter. Get up, put on your workout gear, and go wherever it is you exercise.

Permanent change comes only with persistence. The payoff is worth it. After a month or two, it won't be quite so brutal. After 6 months, it won't be hard at all—you'll look forward to your workouts, your special time to work on yourself, rather than work at whatever your boss or family puts in front of you.

After a year, you're going to want to eat right and exercise for the rest of your life. You're going to crave these things. You're going to hate the days when circumstances prevent you from exercising. When you reach that point, the results will stagger you.

Step 3: Build a foundation. Once you're in the habit of eating right and exercising regularly, you need to make sure your efforts are organized into a set schedule and a basic routine. The workout programs in part two of this book will guide you in this. I'll show you what and how much to do. But it will be up to you to decide when to do it. It will also be up to you to determine your foundation—that is, the absolute minimum dose of exercise that you'll never go below.

Living things thrive on a schedule and a system. The first step in a baby's development is regulating his sleeping and feeding patterns. Can't relate to kids? Okay, think of houseplants. Water them regularly, with steady sun exposure, and they do great. But see what happens when you move them around a lot or water haphazardly. Your fitness program is the same way.

True, life is not so perfect that you always have the luxury of a rigid schedule. But the schedule you put in place and the workout regimen that you establish as your foundation will help you handle disruptions without losing mo-

"Your mindset needs to favor new challenges. You need to seek change, not wait for it to fall on you."

mentum. They'll form a solid place in your life from which you can take off when you're ready to do more, and to which you can go back when circumstances lead you astray.

How do you know what your minimum exercise routine—your foundation—should be? You'll create it over time as you follow the workouts I'll describe, which progress in phases. Just remember that you can always do more than your foundation, and you usually should. Also, you can (and should) modify the elements of your foundation from time to time. And you can and will build a higher and higher foundation as you move ahead.

My way: Set the bar high. My personal baseline is absurdly high, and my schedule is dead set. Those vicious sessions on The Stairs aren't special events for me; they're part of my foundation, along with more orthodox cardio and resistance training, and pick-up sports.

By no means am I suggesting that you set the bar as high as I do. An extra-demanding basic foundation works for me because it means I'm never far away from camera-ready shape. When the call for a cover comes in, I need a minimum of tweaking. Also, when travel or some other contingency throws me off my routine, I'm still flying high.

Same for my schedule. I get up early; share a smoothie with my son, Blaze; brew the coffee; watch Elmo (really!); brush my teeth; and, boom, I'm at The Stairs. If it's my day to watch the little guy, I just carry him around with me. That's 40 more pounds of resistance against gravity going up those steps. Try it some time.

Step 4: Mix it up. The next thing you work on is variety. Your body loves change. Remember, most fitness gains are simply your body adapting to the tasks that you're giving it. Keep giving it the same tasks and eventually it gets used to them. End of progress. But give it new ones and it will adapt in new ways that you're going to love.

The basic principle of muscle growth is progression. To keep getting stronger, you need to lift heavier weights or lift them more times. But I'm talking about more than that here. Besides doing more of the same things, you need to do *different* things.

I know guys who limit their progress because they never vary

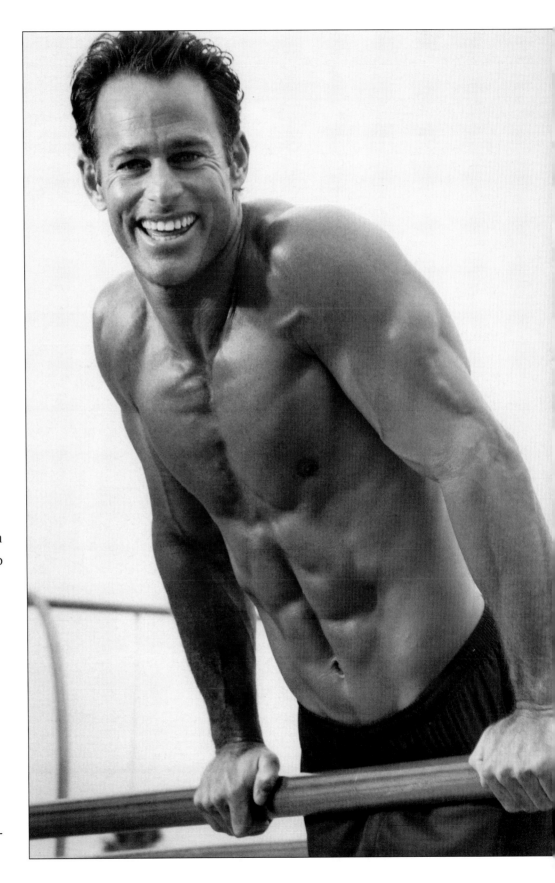

their routines. I mean it; they go to the exact same machine every day and do their 30 minutes (never 29 or 31) at the exact same pace. I applaud their consistency, and they're sure better off than if they did nothing. But they're not getting anywhere near the maximum use of their time. They need to mix it up. I have to admit I've been guilty of the same crime. If I don't make a conscious effort to change my routine, I stay with what's comfortable. That's why I'm talking about the mix-it-up requirement as a factor in your mental approach. Your mindset needs to favor new challenges. You need to seek change, not wait for it to fall on you.

Once you've set your foundation, you should re-tool your program every 4 to 6 weeks. Along the way, make more subtle adjustments, like a wider grip on the barbell or an altered angle of lift. Start rotating new activities into your routine. Get off the bike and on a treadmill. Or swim. Sprint. Play tennis. Give your body new looks and different feels. Whenever you have an opportunity to do something you never do, jump into it.

My way: Do wet workouts. My favorite change of pace is a pool workout. It's not my regular thing, because I can't swim laps for 40 minutes. My upper body just blows after a while, and I can't even move my arms. But if I'm out of town for a shoot and the hotel pool is the best thing going, I'm in there.

I'll give you my pool program in detail here, because it's not in the workout in part two: I do the crawl for the 6 or 7 minutes that my upper body permits. Then I hit my lower body by running in place under water—knees high, heels to butt. That works the hamstrings on the backs of my thighs, the quadriceps on the fronts, my glutes, and my lower abs. Next comes 2 minutes of hard kicking at the side of the pool. By then, my legs are pounding, but my upper body has mellowed out. So I do more laps with another stroke—butterfly (pathetically), breaststroke—and keep the circuit going for 40 minutes.

I burn countless calories and work every muscle in my body. And this workout is something I don't usually do, which means my body has to make new adjustments so that it's ready the next time.

Step 5: Persist, persist, persist.

None of the other elements of my workout means a thing if you're not persistent about them, now and forever. As far as I'm concerned, *persistence* is the most important word in the Cover Model Workout. Only persistence establishes the habits of healthy eating and regular exercise. And only persistence keeps the habit alive through good times and bad.

It takes months to get into shape and even longer to get into the great shape that this book is all about. But it may take only 10 days of doing nothing to get out of shape. Stop persisting and that's what happens. In the long run, persistence is what's going to give you the results you want.

"The biggest favor you'll ever do for yourself and your body is to approach everything as a series of small, doable steps."

Persistence in the short run means getting your workout in, no matter what. Car's broken down and you can't get to the gym? That's the day you do sprints outside your house. Only 20 minutes to exercise? Do it anyway. Hell, I made a video that puts you through a 9-minute workout. Lack of time is never an excuse. Do what you can do.

Hurting? Take it as a challenge, like I do. Exercise the parts of you that feel okay. If your knee is shot, do upper-body work. Don't do anything foolish, but don't let injury defeat you. Persistence.

Maybe it's one of those days when you're just not up for working out. No reason. Nothing's wrong. You just feel lazy. That's the time to deploy your most powerful persistence weapon: your mind.

Ever shuffle along the sidewalk feeling like hell and then an unbelievably hot brunette starts walking that fine walk in front of you? Tell me you don't automatically pick up the pace.

Or say you're practically falling asleep at the wheel when a great song comes on the radio. Next thing you know, you're pounding on the steering wheel and down-shifting, wide awake. The psychological component of physical performance is awesome.

So on those down days, tap into the positive side of your mind to offset your negative tendencies. Think about all the invigorating stuff that goes with exercise. If music and girls don't do it, remind yourself how good you feel after a workout. Or visualize the fat dripping off your body as you sweat on the stationary bike.

I don't care if you suck; just don't quit. Ever. Whenever I compete—whether against other people, an exercise machine, or myself—I imagine that my son is watching me. I'd never want to see him quit, so he'll never see me quit.

Small Steps Get You There

The highlight of my personal workout is The Stairs, a grueling challenge if there ever was one. I do 10 sets of that ridiculously steep 172-step incline, with 15 pullups and 40 pushups after each. That's 1,720 steps, 150 pullups, and 400 pushups—and let me tell you, my legs burn and my heart pounds the whole time. But I always get it done. You know why? Because I take it one step at a time.

Okay, so I actually take it two at a time, but

I'm making a point here. The biggest favor you'll ever do for yourself and your body is to approach everything as a series of small, doable steps.

Getting into shape is nothing but small steps, no matter how advanced a level you've reached. After all, you can do only one workout at a time. During that workout, you can do only one exercise at a time. And each exercise usually consists of a certain number of repetitions of a movement—done one at a time.

The most important benefit of the small-steps approach is that it combats the biggest enemy of your fitness quest: inconsistency. For example, you may not feel up to a 35-minute stationary bike ride today. You consider blowing it off. But you can at least take the small step of sitting on the machine and turning it on. Then you can tell yourself that a 5-minute segment is certainly doable. And the next 5-minute portions will be just as doable. The seventh one will usually turn out to be just as doable. You end up getting it done without changing anything but the way you thought about the task at hand.

Small steps executed consistently get you a lot further than occasional great leaps.

Small steps for beginners. If you're a beginner—or if you haven't worked out in a long time—taking small steps is more than just a mental strategy. It's a physical necessity. Try to pile on multiple sets with heavy weights your first day in the gym and all you're going to get is sore and discouraged. I know you're eager, but start off mellow and work your way up. That's how you create the habit and build that all-important consistency.

"Always do something. Never do nothing. That's how you solidify the fitness habit."

Begin at your own pace. I don't mean yawn your way through a pseudo-workout. But find something that suits you and that will get your heart pumping for 30 to 40 minutes a day. Then find something else that will tax some muscles. Anything you can build on will do the trick.

You know what I consider a super exercise for beginners? Walking. I mean it. For some people, the hardest small step they'll ever take is lacing up some shoes for the first time and getting out there to just *walk*. If you're just getting off the couch for the first time in your life, walking is something you can do to prep yourself before you dive into the actual program I'll be giving you. Walk 20 minutes away from your house and 20 minutes back. That's exercise, my friend. And a very underrated one at that. Do it every day for a week, and then add 10 more minutes to your walk. Throw in a set of six to eight squats at the halfway point. Add 5 more minutes in the third week, with two or three more sets of squats. Then try to include a hill on your walking route. Later, move it up to a jog. You're creating a fitness program in small steps, building up to the first phase of the Cover Model Workout.

Pushups are a great first step as you work your way up to the strength-training part of the workout. Start with what you can do, then build to two sets of 12 or so, 3 days a week. Make it gradual. Remember, you're in this for the long haul.

Same with your diet. Take it slow. For example, I'll repeatedly encourage you to cut way back on what I call the dry carbs: pasta, bread, rice, and potatoes. But you'd be crazy to swear off them completely and immediately. Just try eating them earlier in the day at first. If you have to have that white rice with your fish at night, go ahead and throw it on the plate—but take the portion down.

It's always something. There's one more way that a small-steps mentality will help you get the most out of my program. Don't think of your fitness program as one big monolith. Break it down into the components I introduced earlier in this chapter: cardio exercise, big-muscle weight work, small-muscle training, good nutrition, water guzzling, stretching, and so on. Then accept that you can't do all of them in any one day. But know that you must do one or more of them every day. That gives you a lot less to think about each day. And it gives you an alternative to the all-or-nothing mentality that can lead to blowing off the program completely.

Example: If you can't get your scheduled weight workout in for some reason, don't resign yourself to a nonfitness day. Just grab something else off the component menu. Do cardio. Make sure you eat well that day. Instead of the usual ton of water that I recommend, drink a ton and a half. Or if you're committed to a major pizza blowout because you promised one to your kids, don't just bag your fitness program and spend the night on the couch. That will send you backward twice as fast. Get your workout in before the pizza fest. Maybe steal an extra 20 minutes on the exercise bike. Go for 3 tons of water. Stretch.

Always do something. Never do nothing. That's how you solidify the fitness habit. That's how you build the foundation for taking things to the next level. That's how you unload the flab and pack on the muscle.

My way: Live off the interest. I always think of fitness as an economic system. The individual program components are the currency, and my body is the bank. Every time I do my cardio or strength training or drink extra water, I imagine I'm making a deposit in the fitness bank. If I eat great throughout a day, that's another deposit slip in the old ATM. Sure, sometimes I make a withdrawal. When I treat myself to a plate of pasta at night, I eat into my balance as well. But I'll have made enough deposits during the day to come out ahead.

Now, it's true that I make big deposits. After sprinting The Hill and playing five games of full-court basketball, I'm standing at the special VIP window at the bank. But what matters most is depositing something every day. That's what gets the balance up there over time.

Now I'm living off the interest. I'm burning more calories as I write this than some guys do while they're exercising. Why? Because I've invested in my body. All those deposits have jacked up my muscle-to-fat ratio so that my metabolism won't give flab a fighting chance.

I Know Where the Mountaintop Is—I've Been There

I'm not an exercise physiologist, but I'm always disseminating information about exercise. I'm not a certified trainer, either, but I help people with their training all the time. Nobody's ever asked me for a piece of paper.

If you care, my degree is from the University of Southern California. It's a bachelor's in communications, with an emphasis on public relations. What I really majored in was volleyball, with an em-

phasis on partying. Not surprisingly, I don't attach too much weight to degrees when it comes to training bodies.

I look at it this way. If I'm taking on Mount Everest, who do I want to go up with? A professor who wrote a book on the geology of the Himalayas? Or a climber who's reached the top 12 times? I'm going with the guy who's been there. No contest.

It's the same with getting into peak condition. I've dedicated most of my waking existence to keeping myself superfit and helping others do the same. On the other hand, there are others who have researched lifting surveys and got their degrees for it. Who do you want to emulate?

Guys don't listen to me because I have a certificate proving I can regurgitate things I've read. They come to me because I'm on the cover of *Men's Health* several times a year. Those covers are my degrees. I take that responsibility seriously, and I consider it my solemn duty to provide solid information. What you'll get in the pages ahead is straight talk from the trenches.

All that cover exposure has allowed me to motivate others. I got that exposure by working my butt off to get good enough to represent *Men's Health*. But you know what? There was more to it than that. After all, plenty of other qualified fitness models with great bodies are always around to do cover shots. Why me?

And once chosen, how many cover models get to have a voice, writing fitness articles and books like this? Not many. Why did I?

Something else must have put me over the top, and I'm convinced it was my unusual life story that did it. A guy who maintained maximum fitness with a broken back is good press. And that's only part of what I had to overcome. I know from experience that the story of how I got from where I was to where I am will inspire and motivate you as you start working on a better body and a better life.

So that's what I'm going to get into next. Hang on, though. It's a strange ride.

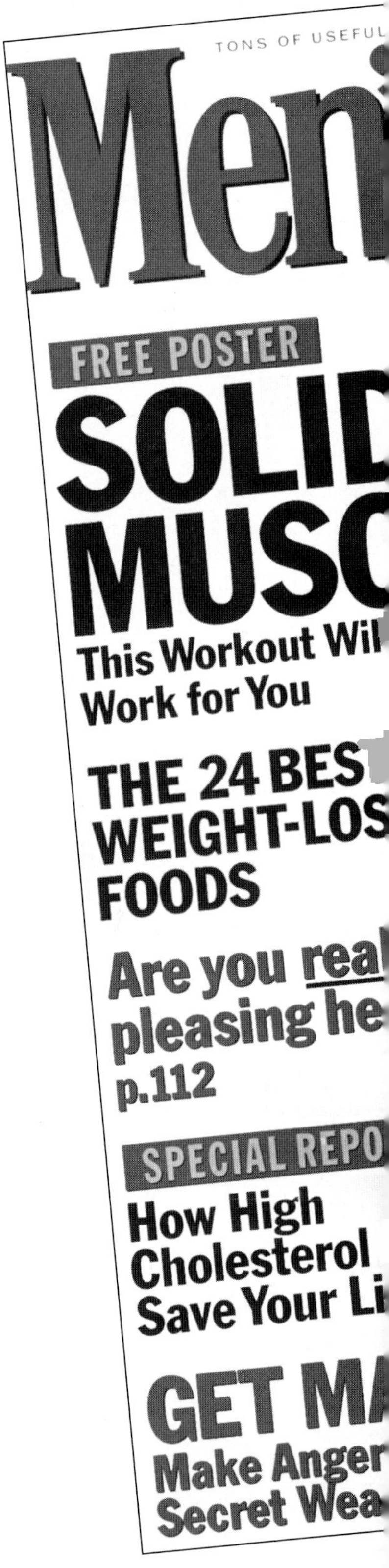

TONS OF USEFUL
Men
FREE POSTER
SOLID
MUSC
This Workout Wil
Work for You
THE 24 BES
WEIGHT-LOS
FOODS
Are you rea
pleasing he
p.112
SPECIAL REPO
How High
Cholesterol
Save Your Li
GET MA
Make Anger
Secret Wea

THE PROBLEM

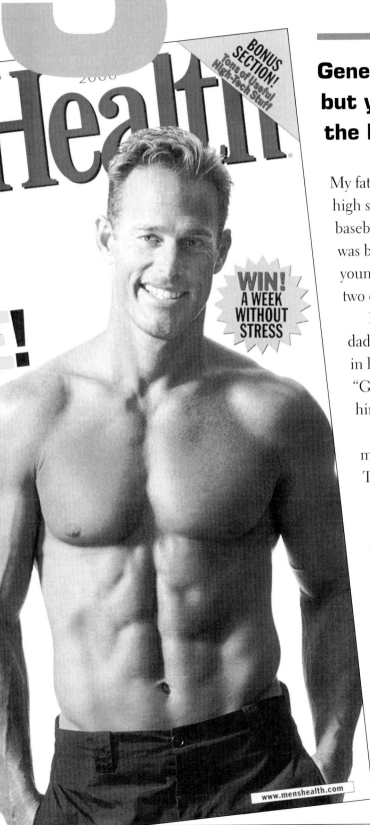

Genetics are a wild card, but you just have to play the hand you're dealt.

My father was George McKibbin: 6 feet 7 inches tall; a high school all-American in football, basketball, and baseball; a marine; the vision of strength and ability. I was born on Long Island, New York, in 1963, the youngest of eight kids. I have five older brothers and two older sisters.

My mom tells me the only time she ever saw my dad cry was when she walked in to find me cradled in his long arms as we watched late-night TV. "George, the doctor said you need rest," she told him. "And it's way past Owen's bedtime."

I looked up at her and said, "But, Mom, he's my best friend." One tear rolled down his cheek. The next day he was dead from a heart attack.

I was 3 years old. He was 41.

His death was a gift of genetics, I'm told. I've spent the rest of my life refusing that gift. I didn't know it at the time, but on that day a source of motivation took shape inside me that would define me as a man.

The Runt of the Litter

My mom dealt with my dad's death by getting as far away from New York as possible without leaving the United States. She packed up and moved all of us to Honolulu, sight unseen. And it was there, on the beach, that I grew up,

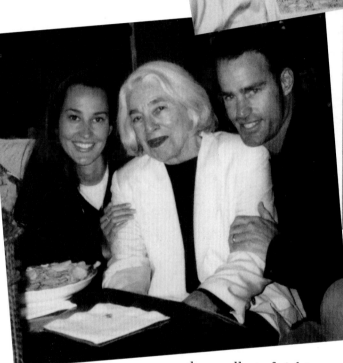

My dad's life and untimely death have been two of the biggest motivators in my life. My wife and mother have been two others.

brothers. Maybe it was Hawaii itself. Whatever it was, I can't remember a time when the racing of my heart from physical exertion wasn't the biggest thrill I could ask for.

I was working out before I knew it was called working out. I hung around my brothers on the beach, trying to emulate everything they did—running, throwing, kicking, or training their lower bodies by hopping down the beach on one leg. I was behind them, the little kid, trying to hop far enough to match their footprints in the sand.

My brothers introduced me to physical power in another way too. It began every morning at 6:00, when I'd wake up and try to sneak into the shower. My brother Angus would intercept me in the hallway, deliver a karate chop to my Adam's apple, strip me of my towel, and hit the shower himself. Hearing the water

the smallest of eight siblings, the runt of the litter.

Mom never remarried. She never even dated. And she never felt sorry for herself, not even when she found out she'd had a coronary episode without knowing it. She just dedicated her life to teaching school and raising eight children, convincing each one of them that he or she was the favorite. If there's a record for youth sporting events attended, she must hold it.

Maybe it was my runt status that got me into all things physical at an early age. Maybe it was the need to defend myself against five older running, the remaining six McKibbins would jockey for position based on age. I get asked a lot what it was like being the youngest of eight. My answer: a lot of cold showers and wet towels.

My way: When things go wrong, I get better. As I got older, I got into soccer and took to it with a passion. It was obvious early on that I had a gift for the sport. I honestly believe that my God-given talent plus my willingness to train like a crazy man could have taken me to the top of the sport.

Unfortunately, I had two other gifts from God: my knees. They were injury-prone, to put it mildly. And my ankles soon followed. Then my back. And my shoulder. Both my knees had a congenital cartilage malformation called discoid meniscus, which was complicated by another condition (in both knees) known as Osgood-Schlatter. The upshot was surgery at age 10 to remove all the cartilage from my right knee. Another surgery revealed the absence of an anterior cruciate ligament in the other knee.

That was only the beginning of my lower-body problems. Since I was so good at soccer, I was playing with young adults when I was still in seventh grade. While that was thrilling, it was not wise for a 12-year-old with knee problems. My legs got very banged up. The worst came when a goalie shattered my kneecap with his head, sending me to the surgeon's table again. I

The eight McKibbin kids with a family friend and two Hawaiian dancers. I'm the runt in the front.

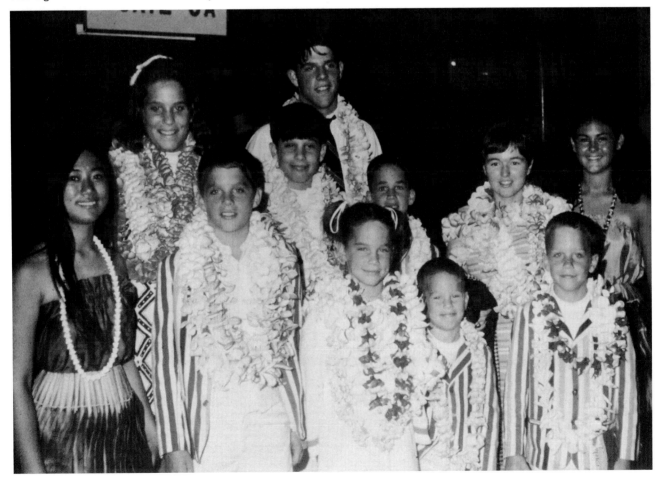

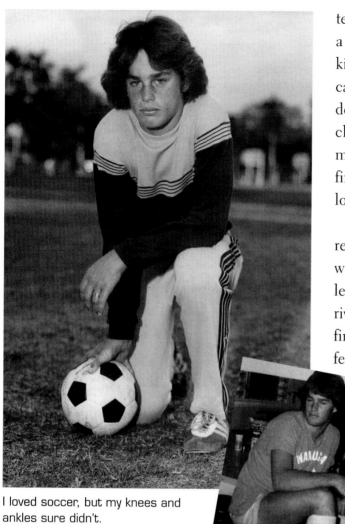
I loved soccer, but my knees and ankles sure didn't.

teenager I was, I created something that's lasted a lifetime. Okay, I thought, if I can't run and kick right now, I'm going to find something I can do. I was curious about weight training and decided to try it out. I had no idea that the muscles I built with weights would one day determine my career path as a model. I just lifted at first because I could, and eventually because I loved it and started to see results.

My point here isn't that I stumbled into a career as a fitness model because of muscles I built while rehabbing from soccer injuries. It's that I learned something important about myself: I derive motivation from adversity. I believe that finding motivation in adversity can make the difference between a cover model body and an average one. This is the single most important concept in this book.

Pain and Volleyball in Los Angeles

My congenitally vulnerable knees doomed my dreams to pursue soccer after high school. The doctor's verdict: no more soccer. Find a sport without so much banging into people.

That news crushed me. I'd never imagined a life without soccer. It was like breaking up with your childhood sweetheart, the only girl you'd ever cared about. It may be for the best, but it hurts.

As you've probably gathered by now, I'm not the kind of guy who lets something like that defeat me. I enrolled at the University of Southern California (USC). That in itself was a major culture shock. Think about it: You've got a

don't think I suffered as much as my brothers did when my mom found out they were letting me play in their league before I had even reached puberty.

The punishment continued in high school, where I made the varsity team as a freshman. My reward was having each ankle in a cast at least four times by my senior year. I ended up spending a lot of my high school years on crutches, unable to do anything with my legs. For a soccer player, that's as bad as it gets.

But instead of moping around like the

Hawaiian beach boy whose idea of formal attire is shorts and rubber sandals. Now, in addition to going to college, he's on a rich-kid campus in downtown Los Angeles, where guys actually wear pleated slacks and pressed polo shirts to class. Let me tell you, it took some getting used to.

As a freshman, I decided to try to make the volleyball team as a walk-on. It was my way of following doctor's orders. Collegiate volleyball is almost as physically demanding as soccer, but there's no physical contact. The only thing you hit is the ball and the floor. I wasn't a complete stranger to the sport—I'd played on my all-state champion high school volleyball team, when I wasn't on crutches—but I'd never dreamed of playing beyond high school. To me, volleyball was mostly something I played with my friends. I used it to meet cool people, not to mention lots of girls. It didn't come naturally for me, like soccer did. In fact, it was a little like teaching my body a foreign language. In soccer, you keep your hands off the ball; in volleyball, you touch it only with your hands.

Somehow, I made the team. And I ended up having a pretty good freshman season— which probably had a lot more to do with adrenaline and physical strength than my as-yet-undeveloped volleyball skills. Also, I hated to lose. That always helps performance.

The last game of the season was against the University of California, Santa Barbara, the number one team in the nation at the time. We'd lost two games and we were getting crushed in a third. The coach put me in as the

"I believe that finding motivation in adversity can make the difference between a cover model body and an average one."

spectators began filing out. I played like I was out of my mind. The next day's edition of USC's newspaper, the *Daily Trojan*, featured a huge article that began with a line from the song "Psycho Killer" by the Talking Heads.

I had broken through and was a force to be reckoned with. I was rewarded with a scholarship for my sophomore year. Southern California was becoming my adopted home. Things were coming together . . . until the McKibbin curse kicked in again.

The Core Problem

At a tournament in Winnipeg, Manitoba, one week before my second season of college volleyball, I went up for a spike and came down on an opponent's foot. My left ankle snapped. Two foreleg bones split. Every ligament in my ankle tore.

Despite these injuries, I couldn't sit out the season, because if I didn't play, I ran the risk of losing my scholarship. USC is an expensive private school, and you don't just let scholarships slip away. So I healed as best I could, stayed in shape while I was recovering, and played out my career as a Trojan by doing all my jumping and landing with my (relatively) good right leg. When I was feeling okay, I played great as an outside hitter. The team was solid. We went to three NCAA finals from 1985 to 1987. In my junior year, we were 29–0 before losing the national-championship match to Pepperdine. (If you don't know what it's like to lose the big one after a perfect season, you don't ever want to.) Without those years on the volleyball court at

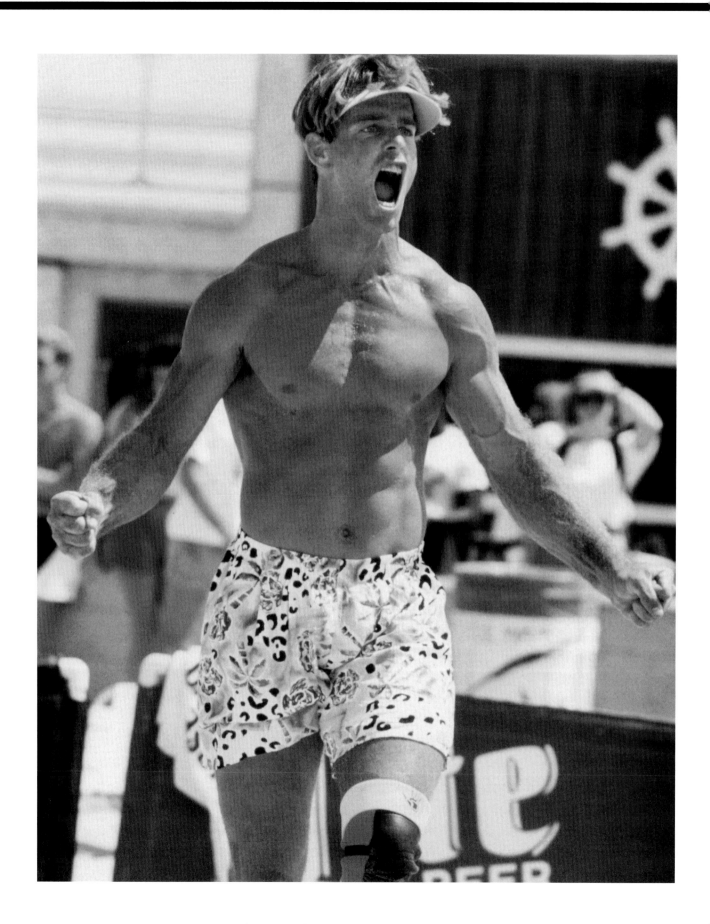

USC, I wouldn't be where I am today.

In retrospect, though, playing on a destroyed ankle was dumb. It forced the rest of my body to compensate for the imbalance. My right leg adjusted by getting bigger and stronger—it's still dramatically bigger than my left leg. At the same time, a sharp pain developed in my lower back.

I was clueless about how serious the problem was. I had no idea that it would haunt my existence for 13 years and come close to killing me. Instead, I'd look around the training room and see every guy in there with an ice pack on his back. I assumed back pain was a normal part of volleyball. So I played through it.

Sand Is Softer Than a Hardwood Floor

After my senior year, I paired up with Adam Johnson, a three-time all-American and Most Valuable Player at USC, to try to qualify for the World Championships of Beach Volleyball Tournament in Redondo Beach. We were a long shot, but we made it in as the last seed. And I guess our collegiate experience on the hard court paid off, because we ended up beating the 11th and 7th seeds before getting ousted. That caught the attention of a clothing company that offered to sponsor me on the Pro Beach Volleyball Tour. The job would involve competition against the top players in the world, TV exposure, the beach as a workplace, global travel, frequent attention from agency reps and talent scouts, and the opportunity to play in front of thousands of enthusiastic fans, a good percentage of them gorgeous babes in bikinis.

I mulled over the offer for about 4 seconds and became a professional beach volleyball player. I spent the summer of 1987 working as a doorman at night and getting my ass kicked playing volleyball during the day. The transition from the team game to the beach version was tougher than my first experience had led me to believe. In case you've got the wrong idea, let me assure you that this version of volleyball is no walk on the beach. It's a grueling physical torture test on hot sand under a hot sun. The court is the same size as it is for team volleyball, and the net is the same height, but the rules are different and there are only two players to a side. So it's just you and your partner in a death match against two savage brutes on the other side of the net who'll do anything to beat you.

As I said, soccer had come naturally to me, but volleyball didn't. I had to work to find my niche in the college game, and then I had to learn the beach game. It was rough. But I mastered it the way you're going to master the Cover Model Workout—in small steps.

That first summer in 1987, I'd be out at the beach at 8:00 A.M. to get five games in, just so I could have my ass kicked five times. Maybe I'd score a point that day. Then the next day, I'd score two. In a few weeks, I'd score seven. Then 12. Then I'd win a game or two. Every day I

"As long as I could function as an athlete, I was going to do it, pain or no pain. . . . I found ways to get around the pain."

I celebrated after a 1994 win.
Check out my mouth—full metal jacket!

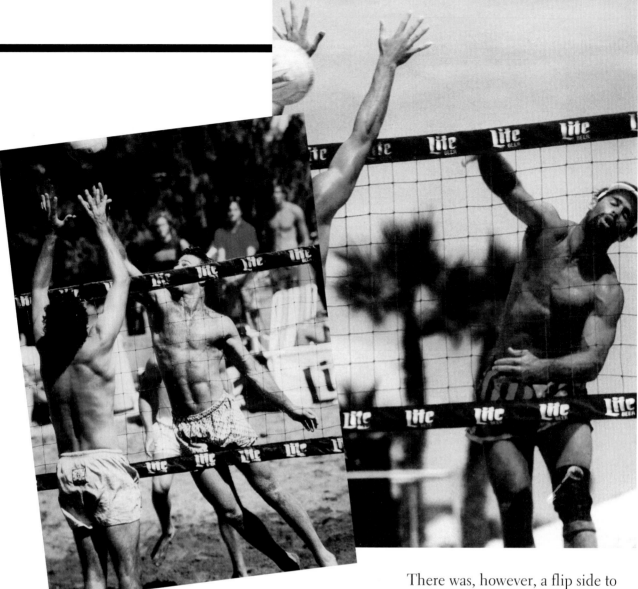

worked hard. Every day I got a little better. Some days it was hard to see the improvement, but I never even considered giving up. By the end of the summer I could compete.

I never was the best player on the tour, but I eventually got good enough to beat the best on a given day. My forte was physical conditioning and strength. Most of the players were in fine shape, but I was in phenomenal shape, to put it bluntly. We played without a game clock through most of my career, so matches could turn into 3-hour endurance contests. The longer the contest, the more my conditioning became an advantage. I never cramped once.

There was, however, a flip side to that advantage: Playing longer matches meant my body hurt more. I knew I could eat some serious pain, but it was getting out of hand.

There's Pain, and Then There's Professional Pain

Beach volleyball is a cutthroat sport. Those guys may look cool, but they attack you like merciless thugs. If you show them a weakness, it's like pouring blood into shark-infested waters. If they'd known about my back, they'd have gone right at it in every match, exploiting my pain and getting a sadistic kick out of doing it. Nothing dirty, you understand, but they could do things like serve me short to make sure I'd spend max-

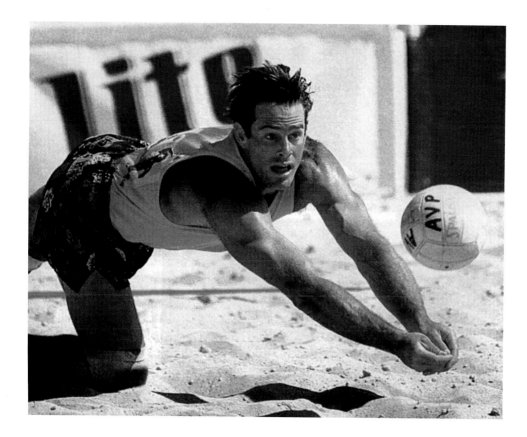

I made a good living as a professional athlete, but I wasn't living a good life.

imum time bending over and straightening up—the last thing you want to do with a bad back.

So I kept my mouth shut. I didn't let on that my knees were destroyed, that my ankle was never right, and that not a day went by without my back screaming with excruciating pain.

Some things I couldn't hide, like the shoulder surgery where they removed ¼ inch of bone, shaved down my rotator cuff, and reconstructed the entire joint. I missed some tournaments with that one. And there were plenty of times when an ankle or knee problem sidelined me. (Weird aside: I spent so much time on crutches between the ages of 10 and 31 that my forearms got disproportionately big and have stayed that way.)

But usually I feigned full recovery, sucked it up, and played hard. I fooled enough people—including myself—to put together a solid career. Tape and Advil can work wonders . . . for a while.

The Worst Was Behind Me

All my other injuries felt like stubbed toes compared to my back. The pain was off the scale. And the worst part of it was that my back hurt like that every single day of my life for 13 solid years. It hurt throughout my twenties and into my thirties. And it kept getting worse.

Sometimes I'd wake up in the morning and want to throw up from the pain. It felt as if a knife were hanging out of my back, with the pain shooting down my legs. It would get so bad that my legs and feet would go numb. Then my chest and shoulders. Even my face. It was unreal.

I know today that my spine was fractured. But the thought never occurred to me then. Who thinks he has a broken back? I figured I had alignment problems and poor circulation. And there was no way I'd give a doctor a shot at it. Word would get out and the sharks would circle.

That sounds pretty irresponsible now, and I suppose it was. But you have to remember, I was an athlete. As long as I could function as an athlete, I was going to do it, pain or no pain. And the amazing thing was, I *could* function. I found ways to get around the pain. When the adrenaline was flowing, I could play like a healthy man for as long as a match lasted. I didn't feel like a healthy man—the pain was always there—but I could play like one. What's weird is that my back would let me do some things but not others—and not the things you might think. I could lift weights, but I couldn't stand to brush my teeth. I could do squats, but it killed me to do the dishes. I could do a bazillion pullups, but bending over just slightly was torture. I could sprint like the wind, but standing still for more than a minute was impossible.

So even with a broken back I managed to maintain my body in peak condition and have a physical advantage over the competition. That strikes people as semi-miraculous. But my condition did not prevent me from doing what I had to do to stay in shape. There's nothing miraculous about working out when you're able to. It hurt like hell, but I could do it. So I did.

Honestly, the pain made me work out harder and watch my diet more carefully. That's partly because of the determination that I've been preaching about. But there were also practical incentives for me to work through the pain.

For one thing, I noticed that staying lean helped ease the pain. Conversely, when I was eating too much, or overdoing the sugar, my back would feel worse. Cardio exercise really helped— in the long run by keeping me lean and in the short run by heating and limbering my body. The biggest relief came from my ab work. I'm telling you, I must have spent a third of my waking hours in a crunch position because squeezing my abs against my spine assuaged the pain. Strong midsection muscles protect your back, of course, and I found out later that my abs and obliques and erectors were virtually functioning as my lower spine.

As I accumulated years on the tour, the gap between my public persona and my private hell grew. The prevailing perception was that Owen McKibbin was living the good life of a top athlete and model with a first-class body. Friends told me I had it all.

I didn't feel like a guy who had it all. I felt like a guy in constant pain. When I looked across the net at my opponent, I wished I could put this unreal pain in *his* body for a change. *I don't care who you are, bro, you couldn't handle this. You'd sit down and cry before the next serve. You'd forfeit. This match would be over. I'd win.*

Looking back, I can see that my back problem probably made me a better person in the long run. I firmly believe in the old saying "What doesn't kill you makes you stronger." Still, it was utter foolishness for me to let the situation go on like it did. My infamous in-your-face competitive streak helped me deal with the pain, but it also needlessly prolonged it. So by all means, follow my workout methods and emulate my discipline. Just don't make the same mistake I did. If you hurt worse and worse as the weeks go by, get checked out. At the same time, take inspiration from the lesson that my story offers. The human body—including *your* human body—has an amazing power to overcome defects and obstacles. It wants to be strong and healthy, and it *will* be if you give it the chance. Even with a broken back, I was able to keep myself in peak condition and perform as an athlete because my body responded as much to my willingness to exercise intensely and my love of physical movement as it did to its physical defects. Though your own obstacles to peak fitness may be different than mine, you have the ability to work through them, just as I did.

As you tackle the Cover Model Workout, never forget that your potential is more important than your problems. Remembering that simple truth allowed me to become a physical icon despite my physical defects. It also allowed me to forge a successful career as a model, against all odds. And that's another story worth telling.

> *"Looking good and feeling good are two different things, of course, and I quickly learned that modeling provided a whole new way to hurt."*

The Very Model of a Modern Major Party Animal

You want to know how a guy like me breaks into the male-icon game? It's not a pretty story. Of course, I wasn't a pretty boy.

Truth is, I was an eyesore for most of my twenties. I'd had my cheekbone shattered, my nose broken a few times, and my lip ripped in half. I wore braces. My hair was long and untamed—on my head *and* my back. I wore a goatee. If you had seen me then, you would have thought I was a total screwup. And you'd have been close to right. Then as now, the beach volleyball scene was loaded with guys with the look that attracts agents in search of clothing models or TV-commercial actors. Except for a few forgettable shots for the clothing company that sponsored me on the tour, I wasn't one of those guys until 1991. Besides my, uh, grooming problems, my physicality wasn't quite on the mark. My body was strong and muscled, and I was in better athletic shape than most of my opponents. But my "big" look wasn't right for fashion or fitness modeling.

Then, when I was 28, my braces came off. I walked around smiling all the time, just because I finally could. My face started coming together, the breaks and tears fading into history. And wouldn't you know it, less than 2 weeks after the braces came off, a woman approached me on the beach and asked if she could take a Polaroid of me. Next thing I knew, I was working with Bruce Weber, a top fashion photographer, for Polo Ralph Lauren.

Not much came of this lucky break, at first. The photos were never published. But a year later, the call came that launched my modeling career in earnest . . . and I did my best to blow it.

As it happened, I got the call a few days before the wedding of my good buddy Joe Myfin. My closest childhood friends had come over from Hawaii, and we were honoring the occasion with a weeklong booze-drenched blowout, which was to culminate that night in an extremely irresponsible bachelor party.

Jack Maiden from the Ford Modeling Agency

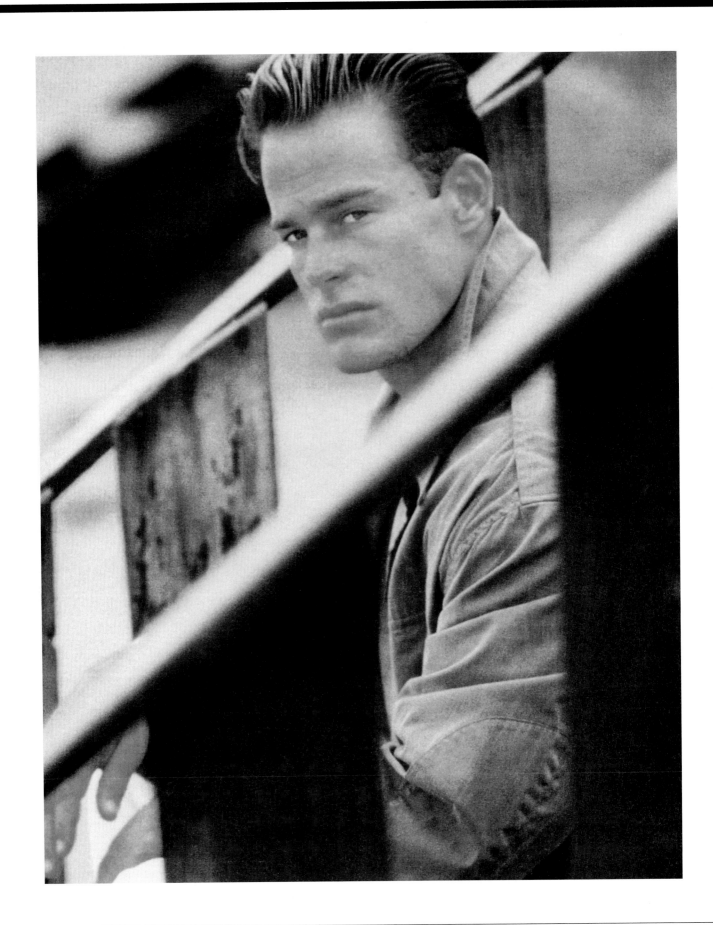

was on the line, insisting that I drop everything and drive over to a Presbyterian church on Melrose Avenue, where a casting for a Hugo Boss print campaign was going on. He'd arranged a time slot for me, but I'd have to hurry.

You know what my first thought was? I was pissed that I'd have to take a real shower. I preferred the beachfront outdoor rinse-off. Still do. My second thought was that I was in no condition to be looked at by people who cared what I looked like. I'd been drinking for days. I needed a shave but didn't have time for one. And I couldn't have done anything with my scraggly, sun-bleached hair if I'd had a week to work on it.

"On the pivotal day of my adult life, the Hugo Boss people thought I was repulsive and the COO of a major corporation thought I was a pervert."

I tried to explain all this, but Jack wouldn't back down. "Just go, Owen." This was a guy on his way to becoming the chief financial officer of one of the most prestigious modeling agencies there is. He was to be obeyed.

On my way out the door, my old friend Ken handed me my portfolio and wished me luck. If this were a screenplay, that would be the moment of foreshadowing when you know something bad is about to happen. Ken, in 50 words or less, is a shit disturber. He's the kind of guy who'll release 500 crickets in his frat brothers' bedrooms. The kind of guy who throws up on a policeman. The kind of guy who'd do anything, to anybody, for a laugh.

Here's my first professionally posed photo, for a 1991 Hugo Boss ad campaign. Notice it was shot from the left—to hide my blown-out right eyeball.

A Portfolio of Blasphemy and Shame

I stumbled into the church looking like a castaway, Gilligan's debauched cousin. I sat, brutally hungover, in front of a somber four-man team, thinking about how far out of my element I was. Later in my career, I'd be able to toss my portfolio down on the table and chill out while my tear sheets did all the selling. But I wasn't a working model yet. I had to sell myself as they flipped through the pages, convince them to give me my first real modeling job. My book was pathetic—not much more than a collection of run-of-the-mill test shots.

At least, that's what I thought it was, until they got to the third page. Now it was a collection of run-of-the-mill publicity shots with thought balloons written on Post-it notes.

"Ooh, that feels good!"

"I'll do whatever it takes!"

And those were the printable ones. My boy Ken had struck again.

I've met lots of very cool people in the fashion-advertising world, but by and large, it's a pretty straightlaced business. I mean, look at the clothes they're peddling. Look at the way they have us posed in the ads. This is not a hang-loose bunch. They take themselves seriously. And these four clients were not amused by Ken's antics, which they assumed were my antics. It's not so much that they took it personally. They simply sized me up as a moron, a screwup, a guy who'd just wasted some of their very valuable time.

I tried to apologize and explain that it had been a prank, but they handed back my book as if it were an oversized turd. When I got home, I chucked the book in the garbage bin outside my apartment. What the hell, I thought, I still had volleyball.

How Far Can a Hard Body Sink?

I got two more calls that afternoon. The first came while I was reconstructing the episode for my howling houseguests. A voice said, "This is A-1 Entertainment. We've got the girls for you tonight." I didn't miss a beat: "But it's only supposed to be one girl." The voice changed and asked to speak to the groom.

But I wouldn't let it go. "Can they do a lesbian dildo show?"

Silence on the other end.

"Look, we're not paying for more than one girl if there's no lesbian dildo show."

Only then did I hand it over to Joe. "You guys order dancers or something?"

Joe took the phone and after a pause I heard him say, "Oh, hi, Dad."

A disastrous day had just gotten worse. Joe's father was chief operating officer of a huge company—and a friend of my mom's. He had made a little lighthearted joke. And I'd sucked the lightness out of it.

So let's review:

On the pivotal day of my adult life, the Hugo Boss people thought I was repulsive and the

"I do hope that my ability to stay with my training in the most impossible of circumstances will convince you what a powerful force for good the exercise habit can be."

COO of a major corporation thought I was a pervert. I knew it would only get worse when I heard from my mom.

The phone rang again. It was Jack, wondering what in hell went on at that church. "Hey, man," I protested, "I told you I wasn't up for—"

"Listen. The client hated you. The photographer loved you. I don't know what you did, but you're booked for a 10-day worldwide print campaign. Sober up. You leave for Mexico City on Monday."

How I Found Out I Had a Good Side

I celebrated by partying like a rock star, which I had planned to do anyway. I got so wasted that I woke up with the entire white area of one eye a dark blood red. Apparently, I'd popped a blood vessel while blowing chow, though God knows I didn't remember it.

So I showed up at Los Angeles Airport on Monday wearing dark glasses—which would have been fine except that it was pouring rain. As fate would have it, I sat next to the one member of the Hugo Boss quartet that despised me the most—the art director who had taken Ken's practical joke as a homophobic cheap shot. It made for an uncomfortable 3-hour flight.

What made it worse was the small matter of my deformed eye. At some point, I'd have to take off those dark glasses. Then what? Twenty minutes before we landed in Mexico City, I hid in the bathroom for a while and concocted my story.

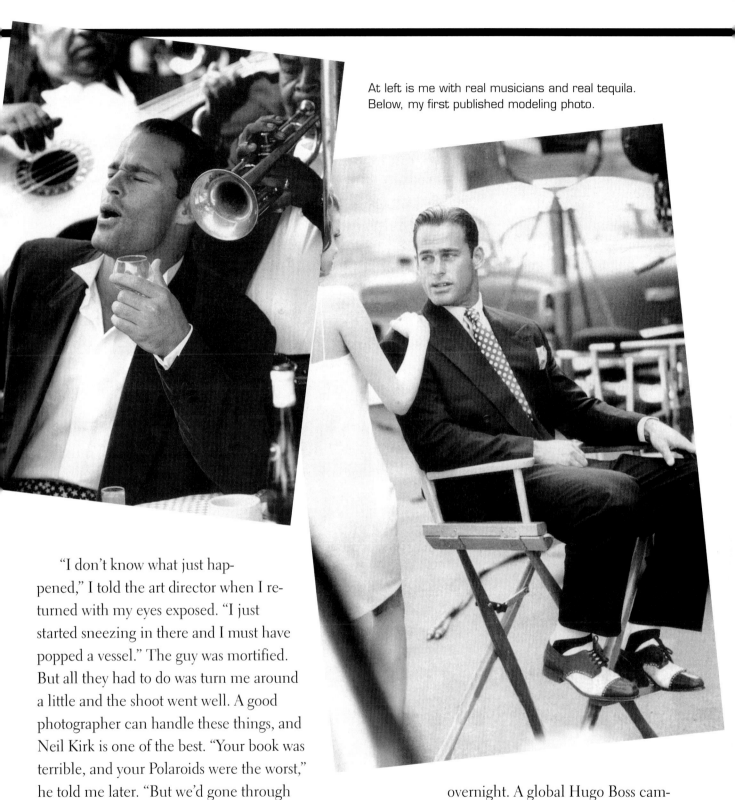

At left is me with real musicians and real tequila. Below, my first published modeling photo.

"I don't know what just happened," I told the art director when I returned with my eyes exposed. "I just started sneezing in there and I must have popped a vessel." The guy was mortified. But all they had to do was turn me around a little and the shoot went well. A good photographer can handle these things, and Neil Kirk is one of the best. "Your book was terrible, and your Polaroids were the worst," he told me later. "But we'd gone through five guys on this project and they were all really boring. So I thought I'd bring you along for a laugh."

I'm still not sure how to take that, but he and I got to be friends. He also made me a print star overnight. A global Hugo Boss campaign is a major deal, the kind of gig you might hope for only after you work your way up for many years. I got it right off the bat.

A week later, thanks to Neil, I was working for British *Vogue* and Guess?, with Claudia

Schiffer and some Victoria's Secret models.

On that shoot, I thought about how in a few months I'd be pitting on the weekends on 120-degree kitty-litter sand someplace, sucking in dust and eating intense pain just so I could scratch my way to something better than a ninth-place finish in a volleyball tournament. Right now, on the other hand, I was hanging out in a motor home with the most beautiful women in the world. While they ran around in their underwear, I waited to go to work in front of the camera, with the photographer and his crew telling me how great I looked.

So This Is What Hell Is Like

Looking good and feeling good are two different things, of course, and I quickly learned that modeling provided a whole new way to hurt. My back never bothered me more than when I was just standing around—and believe me, print models do a lot of standing around.

I'd arrive at a shoot at 8:00 in the morning (sometimes earlier), and within minutes I'd be in so much pain I wanted to scream. And this was while they were still taking Polaroids to test the light. It would only get worse when they were shooting on actual film. My spine felt like it was trying to fly out of my skin. This would go on until 5:00 in the afternoon.

The pain would get so bad that I'd have to take breaks to lie down. Sometimes I'd literally pass out. My eyes were constantly red. And I was always fidgeting, not a recommended habit for models. I must have come off as a head case.

Three-hour volleyball matches were almost a relief. At least I was moving. Physical frenzy was one thing that eased the pain.

Take Two Six-Packs and See Me in the Morning

But physical activity wasn't enough to get me through it completely. Once the match ended and the sun set, it was time to self-medicate. Booze, painkillers, pot—anything to dull the pain.

I got into partying for the same reason any young single guy in Southern California gets into partying—because he can. Especially a young single guy who'd spent his whole life on a Pacific island and then found himself surrounded by blue-eyed blondes and a thousand diversions in the entertainment capital of the world. Between college, beach volleyball, and the fashion world, life was a nonstop party.

But as my back pain persisted, my motive for partying became less and less social and more and more medicinal. I remember times when I'd be walking home with a teammate after practice and I'd sit down on the curb and tell him, "Dude, I can't walk another step. It hurts too much." The guy didn't get it. How could I play volleyball for 6 hours and then not make it another block to the condo 5 minutes later?

We'd procure the 12-pack and commence the self-medication.

I didn't do it lying around the condo like a wino. I partied as I medicated. I was making two incomes and I put them to good use: drinking, traveling, partying, meeting interesting new women. Those aren't necessarily bad things—in fact, they were pretty great things for a while—but it got to the point where I was doing them in a desperate, out-of-control way.

It got so bad that I'd wake up in the morning with no idea how I'd gotten home. I'd go to the bathroom and be amazed that my body still knew how to perform the function. And I'd think, "What do I have to do to you, body, to make you not work anymore?"

But it kept working. And here's the most amazing part: In the middle of all this misery and chaos, I never missed a workout. No matter how bad I felt in the morning, no matter how much pain I was in, I'd always make it to the gym. I'd always run The Hill or do The Stairs. It wasn't always a pretty sight, but I got it done.

This should remind you of a basic premise of the Cover Model Workout that I mentioned in the previous chapter: Exercise must become such an automatic habit for you that skipping it is simply not an option.

That's not to say that regular gym sessions will make up for a suicidal lifestyle. No such luck. But I do hope that my ability to stay with my training in the most impossible of circumstances will convince you what a powerful force for good the exercise habit can be if you force yourself to do what you have to do to acquire it.

And, truth be told, exercise was my salvation. It wasn't going to cure my back or mitigate my self-medication, but it did give me a focus, a reason to go on. Somehow I knew that my body, as much as it tortured me at the time, was going to be my meal ticket, my passport to a better life.

Rock Bottom

In the meantime, I kept up this totally bizarre blend of discipline and destruction. I remember tearing my groin so badly in 1993 that I could barely walk. My partner and I had just finished third in the U.S. Championships. I was to leave soon for the Cleveland Open and then come

back for the World Championships at Hermosa Beach.

I made use of the little time I had between three major tournaments in three weeks by partying so hard that I passed out at a Guns N' Roses concert. Do you have any idea how hard it is to pass out at a Guns N' Roses concert? You've got a decibel level higher than an airborne assault and a building full of thrashing, gyrating bodies. But like I said, I'll meet any challenge.

We finished fourth in Cleveland and ninth at the Worlds—not bad for a two-man team that included a fashion model with a broken back, a pulled groin, and a torn rotator cuff. I was named *Volleyball Monthly* magazine's player of the month for September. The article didn't mention it, but I think I set a record that month for most consecutive vodka cranberries consumed in a 3-week period.

All this seems darkly funny, in retrospect. But those years were mostly dark, with little to laugh about. You wouldn't have liked me then. I was tough on women and even tougher on men. More and more, I wished my pain on others.

My life had reached the crisis stage. I turned 30 with nothing permanent to show for it but pain. I made decent money, but I didn't have a cent. I'd had a million women, but I had no mate. My body looked great, but I was trashed internally and I knew it. I didn't know my back was broken, but I knew I wasn't as healthy as I looked. I was living the opposite of the inside-out, health-first philosophy I supposedly believed in.

When you walk on the dark side like that, your thoughts get dark too. I was heading for a fall. Something had to change.

THE SOLUTION

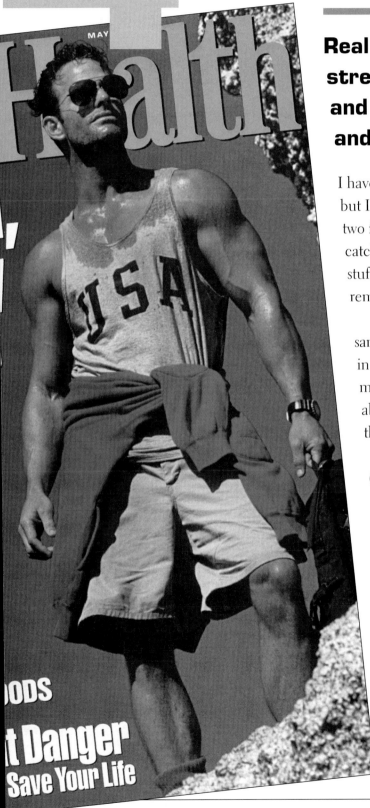

Real fitness means building strength from the inside out— and being true to your body and yourself.

I haven't played any serious soccer since high school, but I can still do amazing things with one ball and two feet—juggle the ball in the air for a while before catching it with the back of my neck, that kind of stuff. It's a great way to warm up for volleyball, while reminding myself what my true sport really is.

That's what I was doing one windy day on the sand in the summer of 1994. For the millionth time in my life, I looked up to scan the beach before a match. For the millionth time in my life, I spotted an absolutely stunning woman walking on the sand. For the first time in my life, I fell in love at first sight.

"Dude, that chick is *hot,*" said my partner. (Yes, people on the beach really do talk like this.)

"Dude," I replied, "that's my wife." Eventually, she was.

I forgot about impressing the crowd with my soccer skills. Instead, I shanked the ball in her direction so that I could throw her the famously strong yet cheesy rap that I'd perfected over many years of beachcombing. I succeeded in convincing her I was the weirdest guy on the beach. She tried to pawn me off on her friend.

She also had a boyfriend. But she had a budding career selling real estate, and that meant her number would be listed. So I asked information for a Lisa Swanson, got that first call in, made my intentions clear . . . and started the waiting game.

The Long-Delayed Diagnosis

Soon after I met Lisa, I went in for an x-ray. My ankle was killing me, which was hardly news. But since it wasn't healing or swelling, I figured I'd broken it somehow. I had. I was sentenced to 3 weeks in a cast.

That should have been enough for one day. But in one of those life moments you find it hard to explain later, I blurted something to my doctor that I'd had no intention of mentioning when I'd walked into his office that day.

"Doc," I said, "if my ankle is broken, I guarantee you my back is broken too. It hurts a hundred times worse than my ankle, and it's hurt every day for 13 years." There. I'd said it. Finally.

Dr. Keith Feder had performed my shoulder and knee surgeries, and knew me well. He thought I was out of my mind for suggesting such a thing. But although he knew my body inside and out, he referred me to a spine specialist.

The specialist and his partner are tops in their field, and I can honestly say they saved my life. They were blown away by my conditioning, considering the circumstances I had been operating under. Still, the first thing they did was x-ray my back while I was bent forward, then backward. And sure enough, there was a break in my lumbar spine, down at the vertebrae labeled L-4 and -5. They were stunned. They'd never heard of anything like it. Human beings just don't walk around with an injury like that, let alone play collegiate and professional sports for 13 years while staying in top shape.

Had I suffered some trauma? Did I get hit by a semi? I said I was pretty sure I'd remember something like that. In that case, he surmised, there was a good chance I was born with the problem.

I'll never know if the broken back was another gift of genetics. The pain hadn't started until I got to college and tried to do all my jumping and landing on my one good ankle. But that doesn't mean the break originally happened then. And at the time, I didn't much care. I just wanted it to go away.

The operation to repair my spine was scheduled in a matter of weeks. I spent a lot of time before the surgery giving blood—to myself. I'd need it to replace what would spill out of me when I went under the knife.

Just Let Me Live. . . .

Being no stranger to surgery, I knew that the better my physical condition when I went in, the quicker my recovery. And believe it or not, I was in as good a shape as ever—despite everything. In fact, I'd made a special effort to be in the best shape of my life for the big event.

Still, I was worried, even if the surgical team wasn't. We weren't talking about routine surgery here. This was my spinal column, after all, not some expendable ligament or piece of cartilage. I found myself asking if I'd still be able to work out when it was over, even if I'd walk again.

"My God," one of the doctors said to me, "if you've been functioning with a back like this, you're going to be running through brick walls by the time we're through with you."

This x-ray finally revealed the cause of my back pain: a break in my spine.

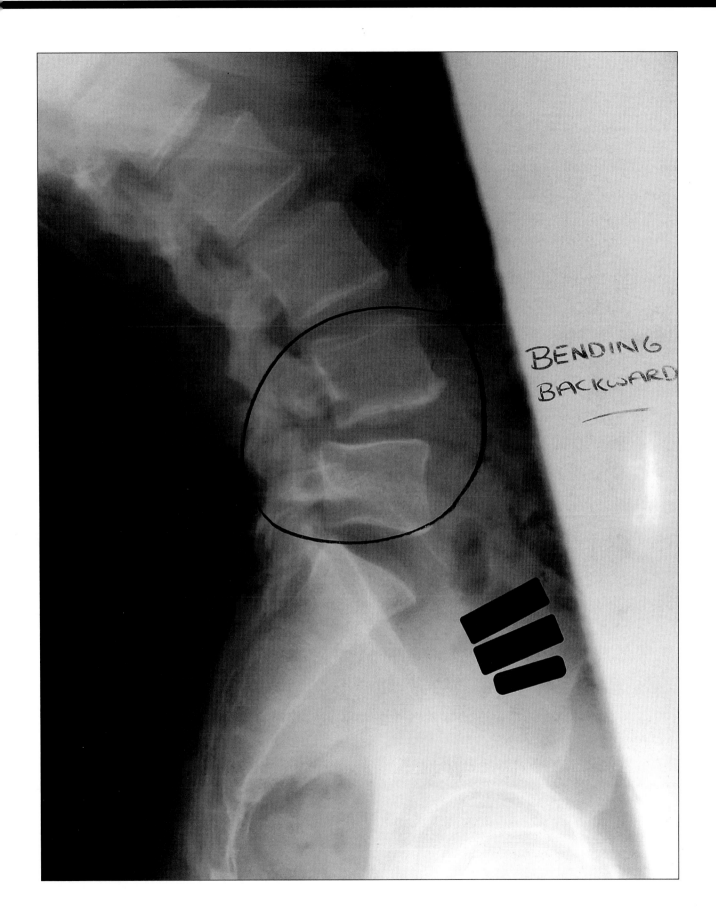

BENDING BACKWARD

Reassuring words, but I still wondered if I would ever wake up once they put me under. I made a promise to God. (I was talking a lot to God in those days.) The deal was this: He lets me make it through this thing, and I change my ways. I lose the party lifestyle. I retire from volleyball, if that's the best thing to do. I clean up my act. And I help others.

I don't mean to speak for the Almighty, but I have to think He's heard that promise a time or two. But I meant it. And I kept it.

Lisa helped me decide to make the promise. True, we weren't a couple yet, but just knowing she existed made a difference. She represented a better life, a brighter future. She inspired me. Hokey? Maybe. But I'm here today, pain-free, healthy, and in the best shape of my life. And she's right here with me as I'm writing this.

Some Guys Never Learn

So what was I doing while the surgery loomed—besides storing blood, making promises, and waiting for Lisa to split with her boyfriend? True to form, I worked out hard and played in beach volleyball tournaments. Nothing had changed, except I now had full knowledge that I was doing it all with a broken back. What the hell, I thought, why not? I'd been doing it for 13 years, maybe for 31. What's another month?

Every athlete likes to go out on his own terms. And the truth is, I played pretty well in those swan songs, even though my ankle was still far from 100 percent and my back still hurt like hell. At least I was cooling it with the partying and self-medicating, by doctors' orders. The main thing, though, was that competition and exercise reminded me that I, Owen McKibbin, was the

master of my body—not genetics, not pain, not any outside influence at all. The motivation I'd found and the discipline I'd developed were still there to serve me. And they always will be, as yours will be as well.

In the middle of all of this, I got the news: Lisa was single again. I called and asked her out. It turned out to be my last first date.

The True Meaning of the Word *Invasive*

On September 14, 1994, I was in an operating room at the Century City Hospital in Los Angeles, where Dr. Robert Bray and Dr. Bob Pashman were preparing to perform a spinal fusion. They had me hanging facedown, sideways over a table, with my knees and ankles touching the padding and my hips and shoulders suspended so that that my upper body was 2 feet in the air. The anesthesiologist had his needle drawn from its holster and loaded with a heavy-duty muscle relaxant.

I was already knocked out, but I'm told that what happened next stunned the entire surgical team. Within 5 seconds of the needle entering my vein, my back buckled and my stomach damn near hit the table. Here's why: My lower back and ab muscles were so strong and hard that they had essentially been serving as my spine, making up for the break. So when they relaxed, the whole thing collapsed. (Keep that in mind when you're doing the midsection exercises I'll be prescribing. You're working muscles that literally hold you up.)

Four 2½-inch-long titanium screws and two titanium plates now hold my spine together.

It's
again.

He
inch w
nally st
hunchi

Clea
Is th

I had n
breakir
God. B
don't g
To be h
no guai
to be al
the drii
wild pa
well-bu

But
have be
with no
would
my recc
didn't w

I di
surgery.
threw a
by an al
a specia
stripper
like an

For
wine ju
self-me
20 glass
was a n

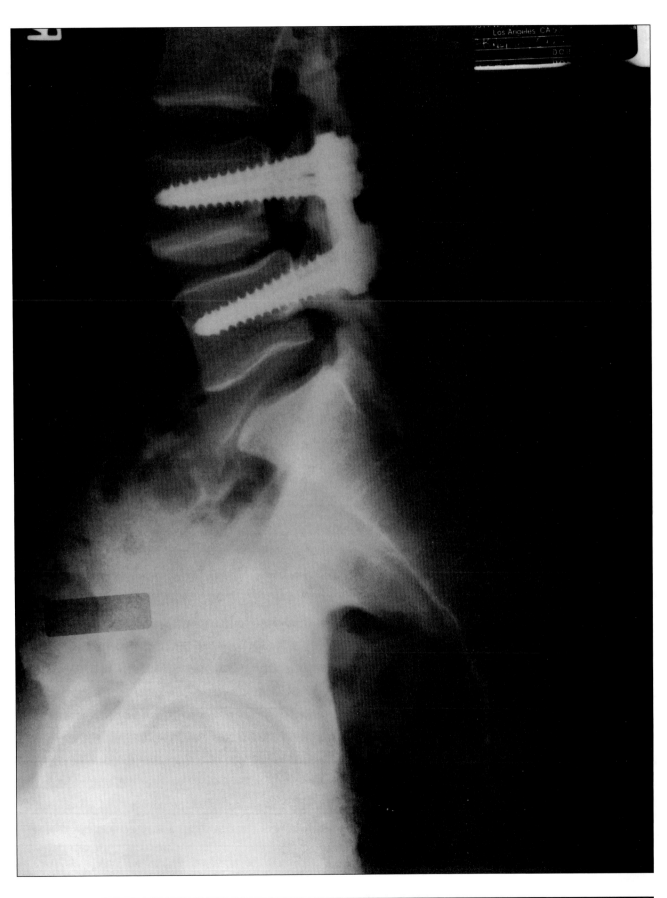

looking for the same things I was—that is, a more grounded existence, a home life, sanity. She wanted to be a better person, and she wanted me to be a better person.

She also made something clear from the get-go. "I'm not going to be one more of your bimbos," she told me. "When you're ready, call me." Her meaning was clear. But as soon as she crawled into bed with me (finally!), I was more than willing to do whatever it would take to keep her there.

That included notifying my female acquaintances that I'd been honorably discharged and would no longer be available for duty. It also involved an uncomfortable confession to Lisa of my wild past. She was going to be hearing a lot of bad shit about me—most of it true—so I figured I might as well lay it all out there.

Full disclosure is a strategy that can backfire on you. Don't try it just because it worked for me with Lisa. I got lucky. Some of what I had to say was painful, not to mention shameful. But she respected me for coming clean.

The way I figure it, there are two routes to clean living. A lot of guys see the right path early, and they quickly hit the groove and stay there. If that's you, more power to you. You're way ahead of the game. Then there are guys like me who have to experience the opposite extreme and hit rock bottom before they get the picture. If I hadn't done all the things I did, I would have been a better athlete and a better

person at the time, but I wouldn't have found the appreciation for clean living that I have now. I may not have had the determination I needed to stay as disciplined as my line of work demands.

I'm a better husband and father for it. What I once feared most in the world—sobriety and monogamy—are two of the most harmonious things in my life today.

> "Probably the most distinctive aspect of my workout is the 'integrity' component geared toward strengthening the often-ignored and usually unseen smaller muscles of your body."

My way: Overcome adversity through motivation and persistence. The story of my life is rock-solid proof that the kind of health I'm pushing in this book is yours for the taking. I'm a living, breathing example of what you can achieve by refusing to allow anything—*anything*—to deter you from your commitment to maximum fitness.

I had no special birthright to a superfit body. Yes, I was born with natural athletic ability and a capacity to exercise more than most people. At the same time, though, I was born with more than my share of physical negatives. Like anybody else, I could have gone either way. Rather than striving to honor my gifts, I could have succumbed to the obstacles placed in my path. But I found the motivation to go for a strong body. And I developed the discipline to achieve it despite adversity. That's the meaning of my life: defeating adversity through motivation and discipline.

I didn't do anything you can't do. You can overcome any obstacle between you and an aesthetically appealing, healthy physique. All you

Here

V
had t
starte
aside
back.
up m
it. M
graft
my h
nium
thick
insid

need is persistence. That persistence is made possible by your motivation. And your motivation is fueled by constantly reminding yourself of the reason you embarked on this quest in the first place.

There are literally millions of American men who would like to improve their bodies but have convinced themselves that fitness is beyond their reach. Or that they're not the fit type. Or that they're too busy, too old, too far gone. Name an excuse, somebody's using it. What they're doing is creating their own obstacles. And they lack the motivation to overcome the roadblocks they've created for themselves. If they're lucky, a doctor will eventually provide them with some motivation: "Shape up or die early."

That's not you, though. I already know you're motivated. Also, you know by now that a better body is not a pipe dream but the logical and inevitable result of consistent exercise and a healthy diet. You know that the body you're striving for is not to be measured against any other body—including mine. The only standard that matters to you is your own inherent potential.

Follow my workout persistently and you're going to learn a lot about that potential. I guarantee that you're going to like what you find out.

Leave Those Genes in the Chromosomes, Where They Belong

I didn't decide to get superfit at a young age in order to be a cover

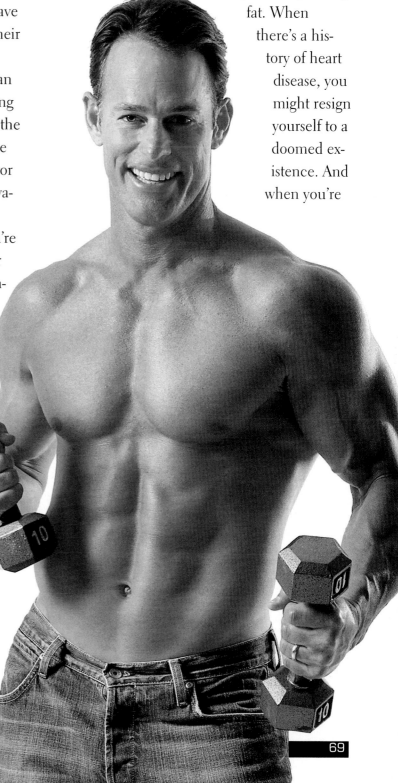

model. I simply set my sights on being as strong and healthy as I could be and refused to let anything stop me. The biggest obstacle I had to overcome was my genetic heritage. When there's an obesity chain in your family, it's pretty easy to accept being fat. When there's a history of heart disease, you might resign yourself to a doomed existence. And when you're born injury-prone, it's tempting to stay in bed for the rest of your life.

I didn't do any of that. Instead, my attitude was basically this: Screw genetics. I'm not going to let genetics determine my fate. No, I'm going to do everything in my power to defeat any gene with a bad attitude. I'm not ever going to be fat. And I'm not going to die of a heart attack in my forties.

I'm convinced that my hard work in overcoming my genetic heritage let me pass along a better hand to my son. Yeah, I know that's scientifically unsound. I couldn't care less. There's no doubt in my mind that little Blaze is a healthier kid because I went after those genes and chewed them up and spit them out.

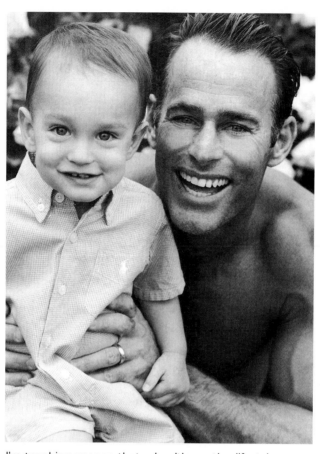

I'm teaching my son that a healthy, active lifestyle can more than make up for our genetic weaknesses.

I truly hope any obstacles you face aren't as painful or scary as mine. If they are, I've shown you that they can be overcome. But it doesn't matter what your obstacles are. No adversity is petty if it's your own. Your struggles are no less important than mine, whatever they are.

What matters is that you know you can beat them. That's the reason I've bored you with my autobiography. I want you to say, "Hey, if that Owen McKibbin guy could do it with a broken back, I can sure as hell do it." Say it out loud. Then get hold of that power within you and get started. You can do it.

The Evolution of My Workout Plan

My recovery from back surgery was phenomenal. I was walking in 3 days. I played tennis 10 days later (which is when I discovered that Lisa plays tennis in a string bikini). I was lifting weights in 20 days. Before 2 months had passed, I was doing a Powerade photo shoot for the Olympics where I had to jump and land repeatedly while hitting a volleyball. Soon I was running and working out harder than ever.

But not exactly the same as ever. The workout you'll soon be doing is the up-to-the-minute version of a work in progress that I've tweaked and improved in bits and pieces throughout my entire life. Not surprisingly, my back-surgery experience led to a few of those tweaks and improvements.

First and foremost, my new emphasis on clean living paid some quick dividends. That's because I was working out harder than before but without having to offset the negative impact of booze, pot, and frequent all-nighters. Do more of the good stuff and less of the bad stuff, and you get better results. Simple as that.

Also, I truly began to appreciate the value of stretching. Like a lot of guys, I didn't have the patience to do much stretching in the early days. But after the surgery, I knew that better lower-body flexibility—in the hip flexors, hams, quads, glutes—would protect my lower back. I really wasn't in the market for any more injuries.

The surgery was only the latest event in my life that shaped the workout I'll be laying out for you. It all started, of course, with my original fitness motivation, which was overcoming my genetic heart disease risk. That started me off immediately with a health-oriented approach to fitness where I would get in shape from the inside out, with no artificial help.

Another key component of my regimen evolved very early on, when I was still a kid. Fitness and sports were always closely linked in my mind, each complementing the other. That's why my workout emphasizes practical development, where you're building muscles to help you move around and get things done in the real world, not just to look good in a tight T-shirt. Is that the approach people expect from a model who specializes in body shots?

"I'm convinced that my hard work in overcoming my genetic heritage let me pass along a better hand to my son."

Maybe not. But it's the way it's always been with me—and with *Men's Health*, for that matter.

Probably the most distinctive aspect of my workout is the "integrity" component geared toward strengthening the often-ignored and usually unseen smaller muscles of your body. My volleyball career had a lot to do with the development of this concept in my workout. People often assume that hitting balls with the same arm thousands of times a day will strengthen that shoulder. What it's more likely to lead to is shoulder injury—*unless* you make a special effort to strengthen the small rotator cuff muscles that control the myriad twisting movements your arm makes.

Integrity training has been as key for me as it will be for you when you dive into the Cover Model Workout. You'll be more thoroughly fit, and your risk of injury will be significantly reduced. Of course, I found ways to get injured anyway. But believe me, I was much better off with my integrity training than I would have been without it.

There was one other addition to my repertoire after the surgery. I did my first cover for *Men's Health* 52 days post-op. The last piece of my fitness puzzle was in place. I was finally cover ready.

PART TWO

THE
COVER MODEL
WORKOUT
PROGRAM

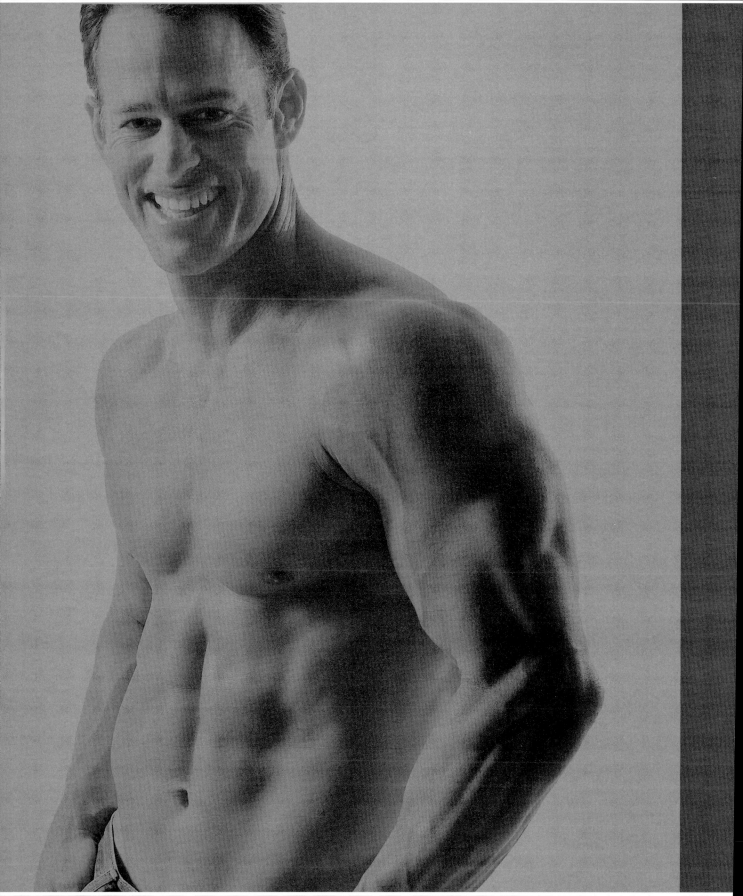

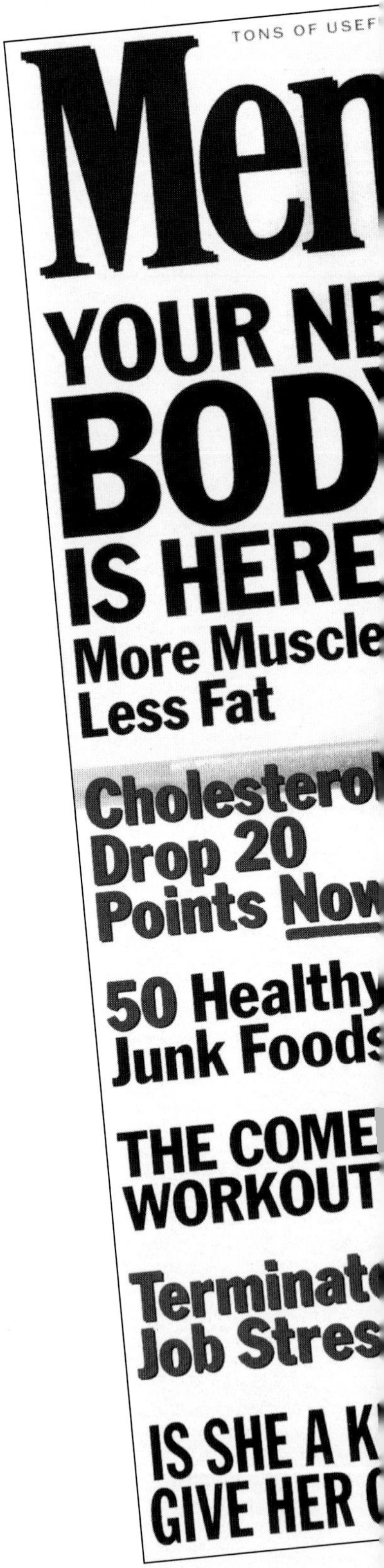

Men

YOUR NE

BODY

IS HERE

More Muscle
Less Fat

Cholesterol
Drop 20
Points Now

50 Healthy
Junk Foods

THE COME
WORKOUT

Terminate
Job Stres

IS SHE A K
GIVE HER C

INTRODUCTION TO THE WORKOUTS

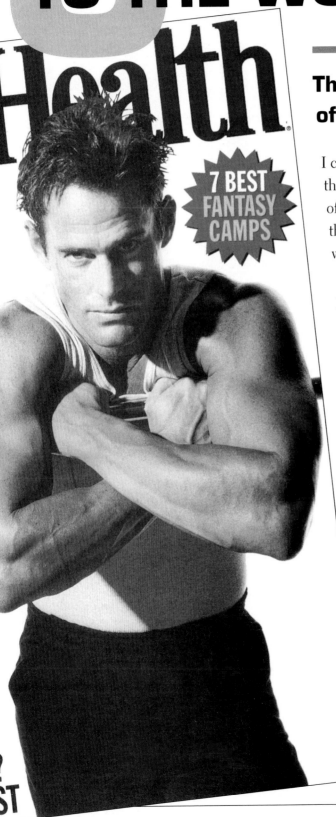

The workouts here are versions of the workouts I do myself.

I change the exercises in my workouts constantly, but the framework described here is what I have used most of my life and will continue to use until I find something that works better. I have no doubt that it will work just as well for you as it has for me.

The weight workouts are based on the concept of progressive overload. You overload your muscles by lifting weights heavy enough to make your muscles work harder than they're used to, but not so heavy that you can't do the prescribed exercises with good form. The progressive part comes from lifting heavier weights as you advance through the program.

In the pages ahead, photographs of each exercise will show you what good form looks like. But I can't tell you how heavy your weights need to be. Proper poundage is different for everybody, and it changes with each exercise.

If you've lifted before, you can use the chart on the following page. It was designed for bench pressers to estimate their one-repetition maximum, or, if they already know their max, to estimate the proper weight to use on sets with higher repetitions.

Here's how it works: Say you know you can bench-press 200 pounds once (that's the sample we use in the chart). That's 100 percent of your one-rep max. And say the workout calls for 10 reps per set. The chart

HOW MUCH WEIGHT SHOULD I LIFT?

Max reps (RM)	1	2	3	4	5	6	7	8	9	10	12	15
% RM	100	95	93	90	87	85	83	80	77	75	67	65
Weight (lb or kg)	200	190	186	180	174	170	166	160	154	150	134	130

tells you to try 75 percent of your max, or 150 pounds in this case.

This isn't a perfect system—depending on your muscle structure, you may be able to do more or fewer reps with any given percentage of your max—and it only tells you how to calculate reps for a single lift. Still, it's a jumping-off point.

If you're starting weight training for the first time, you'll have to use trial and error. If the weight you use is too heavy for the prescribed reps, put it down and pick up a lighter one. If you start out with one that's too light, use more weight the next set or the next workout. When in doubt, start with a weight that's a little lighter than what you think you can handle. If you're correct and it is too light, use a heavier one the next time out. It's better to move up than to start with too much and have to move down.

For your cardiovascular training, the first goal is to build a base of aerobic fitness. You'll work your way up to about 20 minutes of steady, high-intensity exercise. Then you'll move on to shorter workouts of varied intensity—intervals of hard effort interspersed with very-light-effort exercise.

Those are the basic ideas. But if that were all the Cover Model Workout offered, this would be a much shorter book. Here's the other stuff you'll get out of this.

Two Levels

The beginner workout is appropriate for almost everybody—though if you're so completely detrained that you can't walk around the block, you'll need to start with some simple combination of walking and calisthenics, as I described in chapter 2.

But the beginner workout isn't necessarily just for the guy who's never lifted anything heavier than a salad fork. You may want to use it if you used to be in shape but haven't worked out for a long time. It's also a good starting point if you've worked out intermittently without ever sticking with a program long enough to get results.

If, however, you're in pretty good shape already, you can go right to the advanced program. "Pretty good shape" means you should be able to do at least five pullups or chinups, and bench-press and squat your body weight at least once.

If you aren't a beginner but don't qualify for the advanced program, do the beginner program anyway. Then, after 16 weeks, launch into the advanced program. The more solid your fitness base, the more you'll get out of it.

Four Phases

You'll progress through four separate phases, each consisting of an entirely different program. Phase 1 is the most crucial because it builds your first foundation, thickens your tendons and ligaments, and fortifies your entire body so that you can safely integrate the more dynamic movements of the later phases.

Phases 2 and 3 move you up the ladder toward that cover-quality body. Your cardiovascular training progresses through the phases by increasing intensity more than duration. Your biking, running, or cardio-machine work will start to include intervals (all-out efforts alternating with moderate efforts) and sprints.

Your resistance training changes more dramatically with each phase. Essentially, each of the first three phases focuses on different weight-training goals. Key differences in the way you do the exercises can shift the training emphasis from muscular endurance to size to strength.

In Phase 1, The Habit, you'll train for muscle endurance by lifting relatively light (though still challenging) weights at higher repetitions.

In Phase 2, The Muscles, you'll concentrate on building size by fatiguing your muscles rapidly, stimulating them to grow. I'll walk you through exactly how to do that when the time comes.

Phase 3, The Strength, is—not surprisingly—mostly about strength. Here you'll do fewer repetitions with heavier weights.

As you move through the first three phases, you'll feel the gains more and more. By Phase 2, other people will see the gains that you feel. But it's at Phase 4 that you'll really approach the results you wanted when you bought this book.

Phase 4, The Body, gives you a choice of peaking with whatever goal is most important to you. If fat loss is what you need most, you can do the routine in a way that cranks up your metabolism and challenges your body to burn maximum calories. If you're already lean but you want more meat on your bones, I'll show you how to maximize the muscle-building effects of the program. And if strength is more important to you than fat loss or muscle mass, there's a version of the program that works for that goal, too.

This is challenging stuff, and the soonest you can expect to get started on Phase 4 is 3 months into the entire program. Odds are, though, that it will take longer than that.

Never move ahead faster than you're ready. But keep moving ahead. You'll get there.

> *"Key differences in the way you do the exercises can shift the training emphasis from muscular endurance to size to strength."*

First Things First

Here's the most important thing I can tell you about the four stages of the Cover Model Workout: Under no circumstances should you skip Phase 1. I don't care if you finished second in the Ironman last year; Phase 1 is absolutely mandatory if you're going to follow my workout. If you're not a beginner, go ahead and follow the advanced track of Phase 1. But don't start with Phase 2.

The reason Phase 1 is so important is that it conditions your muscles and joints for the specific demands of this particular workout program. Also, remember the foundation concept I talked about in chapter 2? For most guys, I think Phase 1 will serve as a foundation—that is, the fallback routine that represents the minimum you'll do on any given day, even on one of those days when you just don't feel like doing anything.

Fair warning here: Some beginners won't be able to complete the Phase-1 workouts, even on a good day. No problem, as long as you come back next time and try to do a little more. Then, 6 months from now, when you're a master of Phase 4, you'll have Phase 1 to fall back on like an old friend.

Core and Integrity Routines

The strength-training part of each phase is divided into two core sessions and one integrity session per week. It's easiest to do your core workouts on Monday and Friday and your integrity workout on Wednesday.

On the surface, the difference in emphasis between the core and integrity workouts may not be all that obvious. Indeed, some of the specific exercises overlap: You may be asked to do dumbbell bench presses in both your core and integrity days in a given week. But rest assured that the integrity days are designed to strengthen the smaller muscles around your ankles, knees, hips, and shoulders, as well as the stabilizer muscles of your midsection. Of course, you can't do that without also working some of the big mus-

cles, but any redundancy only serves to make you that much stronger. It's a win-win situation.

In general, you should use lighter weight for the integrity moves, especially those that focus on your shoulders.

Compound Moves

The lifts you'll do to build your muscles are, for the most part, compound moves. These are exercises that use more than one major muscle group. Bench presses, for example, primarily work the pectorals, the big muscles that fill your chest. But the triceps on the backs of your upper arms are also big players in this move, since they're the muscles responsible for straightening your arms at the elbows.

Same for the pulldowns that hit the upper-back muscles known as the latissimus dorsi, or lats. In this movement, your biceps also work hard to bend your arms as you pull the bar down. That's a compound movement.

Only after you build a solid strength foundation with compound moves will you start getting into isolation exercises that focus all the work on one muscle group—such as biceps curls, triceps pushdowns, and certain shoulder exercises. Compound moves are more suited to beginners because they really let you feel what it's like to move heavy weight around. And they have a practical advantage because, by bringing various muscles into play, they more closely follow the natural movements you make in life outside the weight room.

I call this creating performance muscles. I don't just want my biceps to bulge or my chest to be big; I want maximum function. I want my muscles to help me take care of physical business in the real world, whatever that business might be. Compound moves help me do that, as does training for strength and endurance as well as for size.

"Phase 1 will serve as a foundation—that is, the fallback routine that represents the minimum you'll do on any given day."

Think Big

Whether the moves are compound or isolation, the core sessions pay a lot of attention to your bigger muscles, such as the quadriceps on the fronts of your thighs, the hamstrings on the backs of your thighs, and the aforementioned lats. That means you'll be working your back and legs a lot more than you may have expected.

The reason for this is simple: If you want your body to have as much lean muscle mass as possible (which you do), it makes sense to work where the most muscle tissue is. That's what will stoke your metabolism for maximum all-day

calorie burning. So think of your legs as fat-elimination engines. When you pound your legs, your whole body gets leaner.

The Truth about Ab Work

I've included a separate chapter to help you get your abdominal muscles into top shape. Still, you may be shocked to see how few midsection exercises are called for in the Cover Model Workout. A fitness model lives and dies by his abs, doesn't he? What gives?

First of all, you'll do enough ab work to get the job done. Don't worry about that. In the Cover Model Workout, the attention paid to your abdominal muscles—as well as the spinal erector muscles of your lower back—is proportional to their size and importance. You don't have to work them an hour a week to build the midsection strength and stability you need.

Time Is on Your Side

The guiding light of the Cover Model Workout is my conviction that intense, concentrated efforts pay off much more than do long, drawn-out sessions of moderate exercise. And that's a definite advantage in this day and age. I don't know many people who have the time for a steady diet of 2-hour workouts.

I set up this program so you'll never have to spend more than an hour at the gym unless you're doing cardio and resistance on the same day and in the same place. You'll do what needs to be done with maximum efficiency in minimum time. That's not just for convenience. It's the best way to get into superb physical condition.

The compound moves I emphasize focus on the efficiency that comes with the short-and-hard approach. You can build awesome biceps and triceps without ever doing a curl or a kickback, because your biceps and triceps do a lot of the work during back and chest exercises. Pullups and pushups are also great examples of combo moves. I'm not saying you won't do any biceps curls or triceps pushdowns. But I am saying that by doing fewer exercises, you'll put more effort into each one. That creates short, intense workouts that lead to quick, awesome results.

I talked earlier, in chapter 2, about sprints being the ideal short-and-hard exercise. The beauty of sprints is you work your muscles, from head to toe, even as you do something that resembles cardio work. (When you sprint, you don't use the energy system that fuels endurance exercise, but you do strengthen your heart.) I also talked about how climbing stairs, as I do in Santa Monica, accomplishes the same thing.

Well, the talking part is over. Soon you'll be doing sprints and stairs—and loving the results.

Intervals and Circuits

The workout instructions ahead look like they favor resistance training over cardiovascular work. In reality, they don't. You'll see a lot more space dedicated to the lifts because there are more individual elements to explain. But the program as a whole strikes the necessary balance. You have to do both.

"The guiding light of the Cover Model Workout is my conviction that intense, concentrated efforts pay off much more than do long, drawn-out sessions of moderate exercise."

I like to think that if you dropped me out of an airplane in the middle of a desert or jungle, I'd make it back to civilization. That's because I've developed, through cardio work, the endurance to cover the ground. And my resistance training gives me the strength to handle anything along the way.

In some stages of the program—the beginning and the end—you'll do circuit routines, which means you'll move quickly from one resistance exercise to the next, with little rest in between. (Not everyone will do their circuits without rest between exercises in the final phase, but I'll explain that when you get there.) This gives you a muscle-building stimulus while also keeping your heart rate elevated, providing some cardiovascular work, too.

Let me warn you now: Circuit routines are no stroll through the gym. In a half-hour (once you work up to that duration), you hit your major muscle groups several times each and suck wind the whole time. It's vicious work. You'll love it.

I'm also going to have you work your way up to incorporating interval training into your cardio work. When I'm on a machine, you won't often see me putting in my 45 minutes at a steady pace. I'll combine intervals of hard and easier exertion.

Patience Is Part of the Program

If you follow the program, you'll make progress. But if you're just starting out, don't expect to see stunning results in the first week or two. Truth is, the purpose of the first month of the program isn't to achieve results you can see or measure. You'll probably notice strength gains, and you'll definitely feel better, but the main thing at first is to build a foundation for the long term. If after the first month you've created the habit of working out consistently, that's the result you were looking for.

Stay off the scale. It would only mislead you. You can drop several pounds without losing an ounce of fat. Or you can shed fat and gain muscle without a budge in your overall body weight. You don't need a scale to tell you how you feel or how your pants fit. And don't check yourself out in the mirror every day, looking for signs of progress. That's like watching a cake bake.

You're going to see improvement over time, but not from day to day. Where you can improve on an almost-daily basis is in the quality and intensity of your exercise. That's where you should focus your attention—not on the scale or the mirror.

If you need to be impatient about something, be impatient to get your workout in. I always am.

My way: Take it personally. You don't last in pro sports for a decade without being a hypercompetitive son of a bitch. I don't know about you, but if some guy starts popping off on the basketball court, that gives me more of a physical rush than any energy bar I've ever eaten. And I focus that energy on one thing: defeating him.

That's the mindset I exploit when I need to. I go to The Hill just so I can look up at it and scoff, "You call yourself a steep hill? I'm going to make you wish you had never been paved." I lay out the challenge to myself: "I'm going to chew up this so-called hill and spit it out."

And I do it every time. I kick that hill's ass. It never kicks mine. Of course, The Hill is not the one puffing and puking when it's all over. But it's also not the one who's in better shape the next morning.

Give that attitude a try as you turn the page and dive into the actual workout chapters. Go ahead and let me have it: "You call this a challenging workout, McKibbin? I'm going to stomp your fluffy-ass program into the ground and bump you right off the cover of *Men's Health*."

That's what I want to hear. Now go do it.

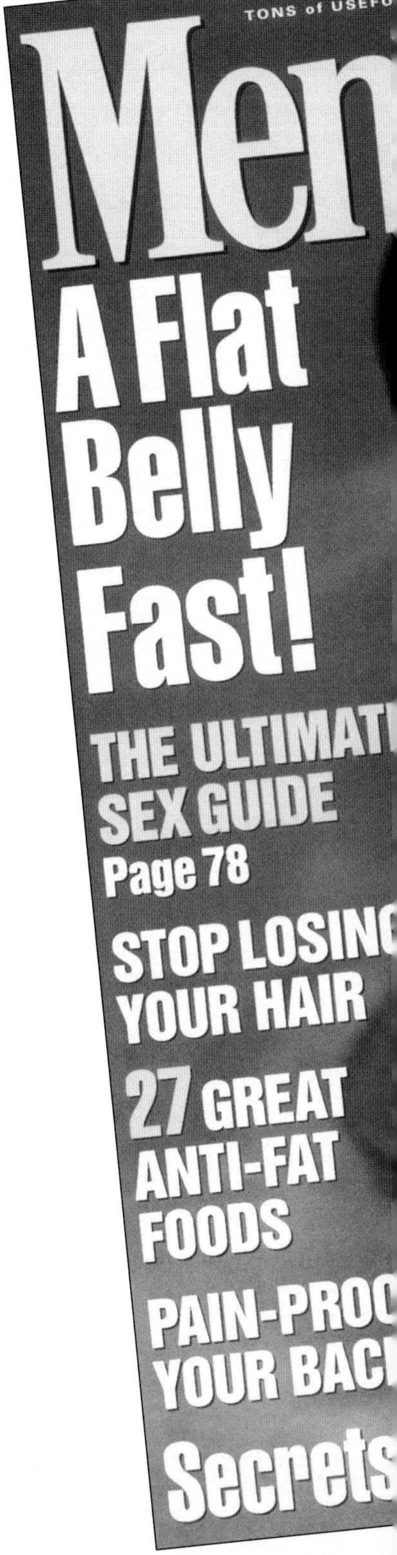
A Flat
Belly
Fast!
SEX GUIDE
Page 78
YOUR HAIR
27 GREAT
ANTI-FAT
FOODS

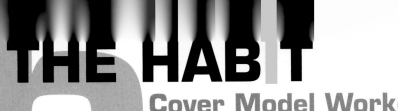

THE HABIT
Cover Model Workout, **Phase 1**

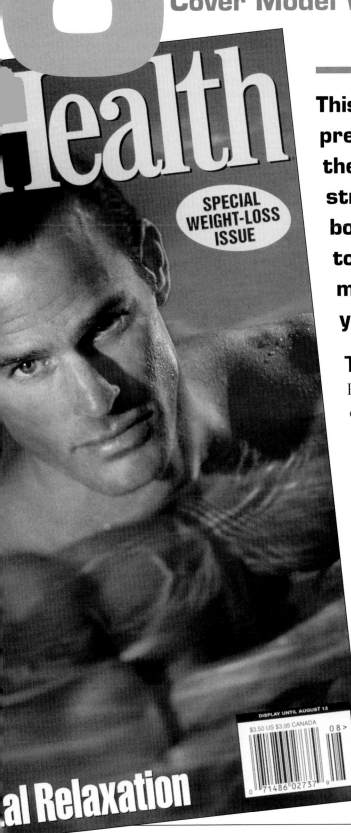

This 4-week program prepares your body for the heavy muscle-enhancing, strength-building, and body-changing workouts to come. That doesn't mean it's easy—if it is, you're doing something wrong.

The Goals

Physically, Phase 1 develops muscle endurance and connective-tissue strength, increases muscle mass (although the next phase will do that in a much more dramatic way), and, perhaps most important, gets your body used to doing strenuous exercise three times a week.

Psychologically, this should be your default routine. For the rest of your life, on any regular workout day when you feel unmotivated and tempted to blow off your exercise session, I want you to go to your gym or home-workout area and do this routine. I want this to be the bare minimum of exercise you accept from yourself on your workout days.

The Routines

As in all four phases of the Cover Model Workout, you'll do three weight workouts each week. You'll do the core routine twice (preferably Monday and Friday) and the integrity routine once (Wednesday, most likely).

Core routine: The core routine in this chapter works all your major muscles with the idea of achieving big improvements in muscle endurance, substantial improvements in muscle size, and modest improvements in strength.

Integrity routine: This month, the integrity routine works all your muscles but puts special emphasis on the ones you're most likely to injure early in a weight-training program. In my experience, guys tend to tweak their shoulders first. Those are the most mobile joints on the body, and although they're capable of generating a lot of force, they also offer lots of opportunity to pull, twist, pinch, or inflame a variety of muscles and connective tissues. In the integrity routine, I've included two chest-and-shoulder exercises to increase the stability of the shoulders' connective tissues and the endurance of their muscle fibers.

Between the core and integrity routines, you'll end up working your chest and shoulder muscles three times a week. That may seem like a lot—especially if you have been lifting for a few years and have gotten into routines that work major muscle groups just once or twice a week. But I have my reasons. My major goal with these low-weight, high-repetition routines is to improve your muscle endurance and connective-tissue strength while giving you the first hint of the increases in muscle size you'll achieve in the Cover Model Workout. When the weights get heavier and the repetitions get fewer, you won't work major muscles three times a week.

Beginner versus Advanced

Look, I know nobody wants to consider himself a beginner. So I want to take the negative connotations out of the word. As I explained in the previous chapter, in these routines, a beginner is someone who hasn't worked out before, hasn't worked out in a long time, has worked out only haphazardly, or hasn't worked out successfully.

Advanced, on the other hand, may be too big a word for what I expect here. The first definition of advanced is someone who has been training for at least a few months consecutively and has gotten noticeably stronger, bigger, or leaner.

A second definition is a guy who can do at least five pullups or chinups, and bench-press and squat his body weight at least once.

If the second definition fits you even though the first does not, do the advanced routine anyway. However, if you qualify under the first definition but you still can't do a pullup and have never before done squats, I think you'll be better off doing the beginner routine, completing it, and then starting over with the advanced program.

Time

You should finish all your workouts—beginner or advanced—in well under an hour.

Warmup

You don't have to knock yourself out on the warmups when you're doing high-repetition weight routines. Still, you need to do something to prepare your body for hard work.

Beginners could do 5 minutes of a general warmup—5 minutes on a treadmill or exercise bike, or calisthenics, if you're working out at home. Or you could do the entire circuit of exercises in the workouts, using less weight than you'll use in the actual workout. So if you plan to do 12 to 15 repetitions of wide-grip lat pulldowns with 40 pounds in the workout, you could do 10 repetitions with 30 pounds in your warmup circuit. Remember, a warmup set should never take your muscles to a point of exhaustion. Save that for the actual workout.

For advanced guys, it's a good idea to do one or

two warmup sets of the first lower-body and first upper-body exercises in each workout. Doing so will lubricate your joints and prepare your lower- and upper-body motor units for the specific movements. So let's say you're going to do a work set of 20 squats with 135 pounds, followed immediately by a drop set of 10 reps with 95 pounds. You might first do a warmup set of 10 reps with 95, rest for 30 seconds, then do a second warmup set of 5 with 135. Rest for a minute, then do your two work sets.

> *"You're going to see improvement over time, but not from day to day. Where you can improve on an almost-daily basis is in the quality and intensity of your exercise."*

Speed

You want to perform repetitions deliberately. Your natural instinct may be to raise the weights in 1 second and lower them in 2. I want you to lift more slowly than your instincts say you should— maybe 2 seconds to raise the weight, and 3 or 4 seconds to lower it.

Here's a simple way to force yourself to lift more slowly: Pause at both ends of the lift—in the fully contracted position, and when you've lowered the weight and are ready to begin the next repetition. If you pause after lifting the weights in a dumbbell bench press, for example, you keep tension on your chest and shoulder muscles a bit longer, and that can also help strengthen your connective tissues. If you pause after lowering the weights, you take momentum out of the lift, forcing your muscles to work harder at the beginning of each repetition.

One caution: When you pause, don't

release tension on your muscles. That can lead to sloppy form and less muscle-growth stimulus.

Rest between Exercises

In both the advanced and beginner routines, try to keep rest to 30 seconds or less. You may not be able to pull that off, especially if you're exercising at home and you can't change the weights that quickly to prepare for the next exercise. In that case, just move as fast as you can between exercises.

Cardiovascular Routine

I'll give you detailed instructions after each weight routine. Here, you just need to decide when you're going to do your cardio work. I want you to do three cardio workouts a week. You can do them after your weight workouts or on separate days.

Don't do your cardio routine before you lift. You can have a good cardio workout following a strength routine, but the converse isn't true. You need to be fresh to hit the weights with the kind of intensity that delivers results. If you do the aerobic work first, you run the risk of depleting your muscles of the fuel they need for lifting, and of raising your core temperature to a degree at which your muscles can't work efficiently and productively.

Beginner Routine

CORE WORKOUT: MONDAYS AND FRIDAYS

Exercise	Reps	Week 1	Week 1	Week 2	Week 2	Week 3	Week 3	Week 4	Week 4
		Weight/Reps	Weight/Reps	Weight/Reps	Weight/Reps	Weight/Reps	Weight/Reps	Weight/Reps	Weight/Reps
Squat	12–15								
Wide-grip lat pulldown	12–15								
Neutral-grip lat pulldown	12–15								
Lying leg curl	12–15								
Dumbbell bench press	12–15								
Dumbbell shoulder press	12–15								
Superman	12–15								
Owen crunch	12–15								

INTEGRITY WORKOUT: WEDNESDAYS

Exercise	Reps	Week 1	Week 2	Week 3	Week 4
		Weight/Reps	Weight/Reps	Weight/Reps	Weight/Reps
Dumbbell bench press	12–15				
Pushup	12–15*				
Dumbbell shoulder press	12–15				
Seated lateral raise	12–15				
Walking lunge	12–15				
Overhand-grip machine row	12–15				
Owen crunch	12–15				

* If you can't do 12–15, just do as many as you can.

Cardiovascular-Training Workout

Do your cardiovascular training either immediately after your resistance-training workout or on your days off. If you haven't done any cardiovascular exercise in the past 6 months, or if you're more than 15 pounds overweight, start out by walking or riding a bike (or stationary cycle) for 10 to 15 minutes. If you walk on a treadmill, set it on a slight incline (2 to 5 degrees); if you don't use an incline, it's easier than walking outdoors. The intensity doesn't matter, especially in the first week. You should always finish your cardiovascular exercise feeling that you could've done more. Try to go about 10 percent longer each week. Or go a little harder in the same amount of time—increase the incline or speed of the treadmill, for example.

RATING YOUR CARDIO EFFORT

Perceived Exertion	How Hard?	Breathing	Can You Talk?	% Maximum Effort
1	Very easy	Normal	Until someone interrupts	35
2	Easy	Still normal	"As I was saying, . . ."	45
3	Light, but starting to feel like exercise	Comfortable	No problem yet	55
4	Somewhat hard	Noticeably deeper	Possible, but no soliloquies	65
5	Hard	Deep but steady	Just name, rank, and serial number	75
6	Between hard and very hard	Deep and getting faster	Name only	85
7	Very hard	Deep and fast	Initials only	90
8	Very, very hard	Very deep and very fast	Maybe a grunt	95
9	So hard you can do it for only a few seconds	Panting	A gasp	97.5
10	Maximum effort	Can't breathe	Can't even gasp	100

Advanced Routine

Drop Sets

Drop sets crank up mechanisms linked to both muscle building and fat burning. Do a set of the designated repetitions (10 or 20) with a weight you consider challenging. By the time you get to the final repetition, you should feel that your muscles are right at the point of exhaustion. Immediately put down the weight and select another that's about 20 percent lighter. Do 10 repetitions with that weight.

Say you do 20 squats with 135 pounds (a 7-foot Olympic barbell—that's the big one—with a 45-pound plate on each side). After you finish, pull off the 45s and put on a pair of 25-pound plates and a pair of 5s.

CORE WORKOUT: MONDAYS AND FRIDAYS

Exercise	Reps	Week 1	Week 1	Week 2	Week 2	Week 3	Week 3	Week 4	Week 4
		Weight/Reps	Weight/Reps	Weight/Reps	Weight/Reps	Weight/Reps	Weight/Reps	Weight/Reps	Weight/Reps
Squat									
Set 1	20								
Set 2 (drop)	10								
Wide-grip lat pulldown									
Set 1	10								
Set 2 (drop)	10								
Neutral-grip lat pulldown									
Set 1	10								
Set 2 (drop)	10								
Lying leg curl									
Set 1	10								
Set 2 (drop)	10								
Dumbbell bench press	8–10								
Dumbbell shoulder press	8–10								
Superman	12–15								
Owen crunch	12–15								

INTEGRITY WORKOUT: WEDNESDAYS

Exercise	Reps	Week 1	Week 2	Week 3	Week 4
		Weight/Reps	Weight/Reps	Weight/Reps	Weight/Reps
Dumbbell bench press					
Set 1	10				
Set 2 (drop)	10				
Pushup	20				
Dumbbell shoulder press					
Set 1	10				
Set 2 (drop)	10				
Seated lateral raise					
Set 1	10				
Set 2 (drop)	10				
Walking lunge	8–10				
Overhand-grip machine row	8–10				
Owen crunch	12–15				

Cardiovascular-Training Workout

If you've been doing cardiovascular exercise consistently for the past 6 months, try this 20-minute, high-intensity interval routine. It'll prepare you for the more difficult interval routines in the next three phases. And since high-intensity training stimulates your body to keep burning calories even after you finish exercising, you'll increase your metabolism after just one workout.

Perform each sprint described at right on a treadmill or an exercise bike at the prescribed percentage of your highest possible effort (see "Rating Your Cardio Effort" on page 88 to determine each percentage). Then, slow to an active rest at a lower intensity—a light jog, for instance.

Warm up for 5 minutes, gradually increasing your intensity to about 50 percent of full effort.

→ Sprint for 30 seconds at 85 percent of full effort.

→ Take an active rest for 2 minutes at 45 percent of full effort.

→ Sprint for 20 seconds at 90 percent of full effort.

→ Take an active rest for 2 minutes at 45 percent of full effort.

→ Sprint for 10 seconds at 100 percent (full sprint).

→ Take an active rest for 2 minutes at 45 percent of full effort.

→ Sprint for 20 seconds at 90 percent of full effort.

→ Take an active rest for 2 minutes at 45 percent of full effort.

→ Sprint for 30 seconds at 85 percent of full effort.

→ Cool down for 5 minutes.

"Never forget that the habit is a baseline. It's the minimum you have to do to maintain your health-and-fitness foundation."

The Exercises

SQUAT

1 Set a barbell on a squat rack and step under it so the bar rests across your upper back. Pull your shoulders back as you grab the bar with an overhand grip. The bar should sit comfortably on your upper trapezius muscles. Lift the bar off the rack and step back. Set your feet shoulder-width apart, and keep your knees slightly bent, your back straight, and your eyes focused straight ahead.

2 Slowly lower your body as if you were sitting back into a chair, keeping your back in its natural alignment and your lower legs nearly perpendicular to the floor. When your thighs are parallel to the floor, pause. Then return to the starting position.

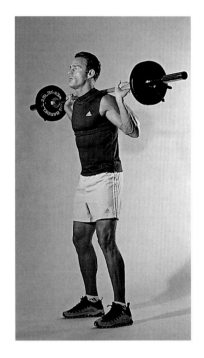
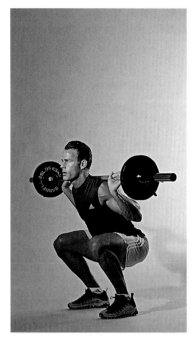

WIDE-GRIP LAT PULLDOWN

1 Attach a long bar to the high pulley of a pulldown machine. Sit upright in the machine and grab the bar with a wide, overhand grip.

2 Pull the bar down to your chest without leaning backward more than a few degrees. (It works best when you try to push your chest up to meet the bar, instead of simply pulling the bar down to your chest.) Pause, then slowly return to the starting position.

If you don't have access to this machine: Do a pullover with dumbbells. Lie faceup on a bench and hold the weights over your chest with your arms extended, your elbows slightly bent, and your palms facing your toes. The weights should be perpendicular to the floor. Keeping your back flat against the bench to elongate your lats, slowly lower the weights behind your head until your upper arms are parallel to the floor. Then pull the weights back to the starting position. Keep a slight bend in your elbows throughout.

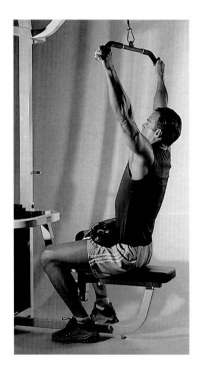
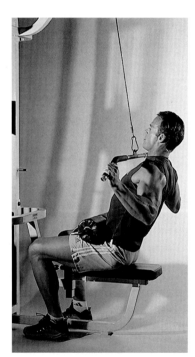

NEUTRAL-GRIP LAT PULLDOWN

1 Attach the parallel-grip handle to the lat-pulldown cable. Grab the handle with an overhand grip so your palms face each other. Sit, positioning your knees under the pad.

2 Pull the handle down to your chest. Pause, then slowly return to the starting position.

If you don't have access to this machine: Do the pullover described as an alternative to the wide-grip lat pulldown, but hold the dumbbells as close together as possible, with your palms facing each other.

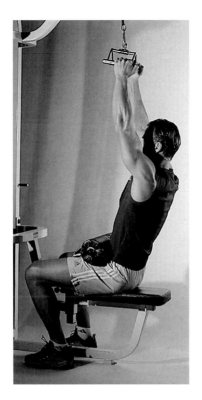 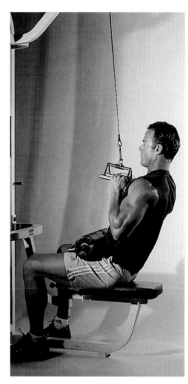

LYING LEG CURL

1 Lie on the leg-curl machine with the pads against your lower legs, above your heels and below your calf muscles.

2 Without raising your hips off the bench, bend your knees to pull the weight toward your butt as far as you can. Pause, then slowly return to the starting position.

If you don't have access to this machine: Do the exercise lying on a bench, holding a dumbbell between your feet.

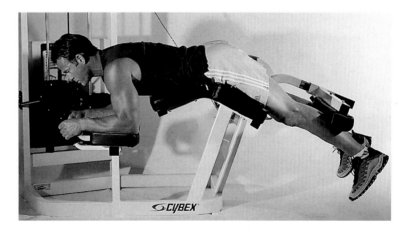

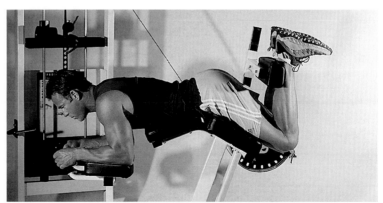

DUMBBELL BENCH PRESS

1 Grab a pair of dumbbells and lie faceup on a flat bench. Hold the dumbbells just outside your shoulders, with your arms bent and your palms facing your feet.

2 Push the weights up and slightly inward so that when your arms are extended, the dumbbells are above your collarbones. Lower the weights back to your chest, and pause before repeating.

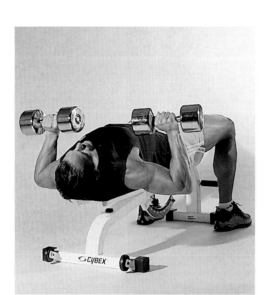
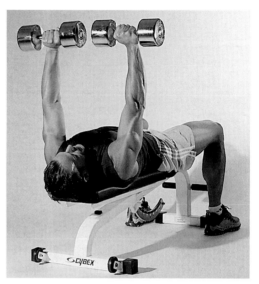

DUMBBELL SHOULDER PRESS

1 Grab a pair of dumbbells and sit holding them just outside your shoulders, with your arms bent and your palms facing each other.

2 Push the weights straight overhead. Pause, then slowly lower them.

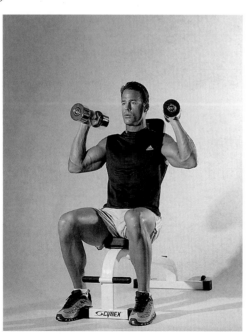
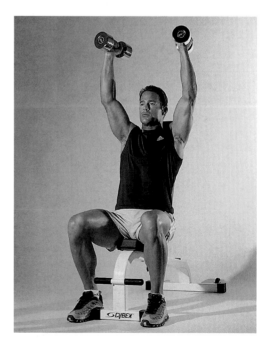

SUPERMAN

1 Lie facedown on the floor with your arms extended above your head, palms down.

2 Lift your head, chest, arms, thighs, and lower legs off the floor as high as possible. Pause, then return to the starting position.

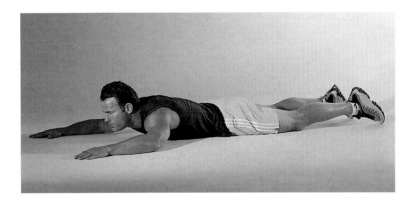

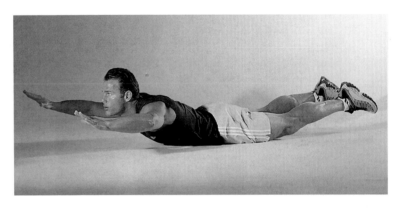

PUSHUP

1 Position yourself facedown on the floor, with your weight supported on your hands and toes. Your hands should be shoulder-width apart, fingers pointed forward. Your feet should be hip-width apart. Keep your arms, back, and legs straight.

2 Bend at the elbows to slowly lower yourself to the floor. Stop when your chest is an inch from the floor, pause, then push yourself back up to the starting position.

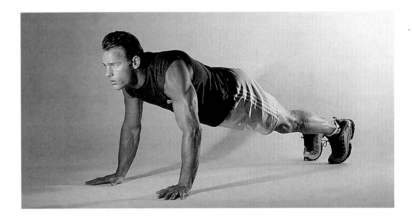

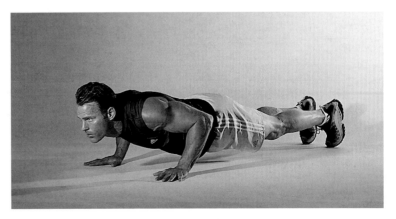

SEATED LATERAL RAISE

1 Sit holding a pair of dumbbells at arm's length with your palms turned toward each other. Start with your elbows bent slightly and your arms at about a 30-degree angle with your torso. (From zero to about 30 degrees is "free" space; your arms can move the weights to this point with no effort. So simply start at the point at which the exercise is difficult.)

2 Without changing the bend in your elbows, raise your arms out to the sides until they're parallel to the floor. Pause, then lower them back to the starting position.

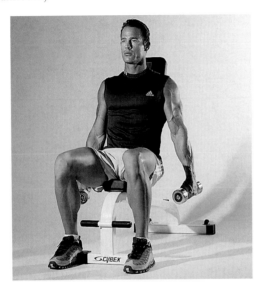

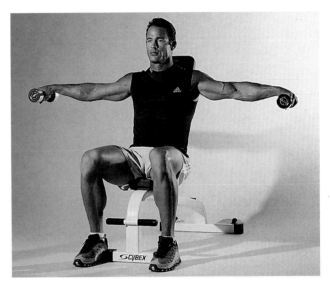

WALKING LUNGE

1 Grab a pair of dumbbells and hold them at your sides. Stand with your feet hip-width apart at one end of your house or gym.

2 Lunge forward with your nondominant leg (your left if you're right-handed), bending your knee 90 degrees. Your other knee should also bend and almost touch the floor.

Stand and bring your back foot up next to your front foot, then repeat with your dominant leg lunging forward. That's one repetition. Continue until you've completed half of your repetitions in this direction. Then turn and do the same number of walking lunges back to your starting point.

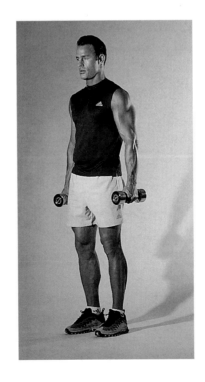

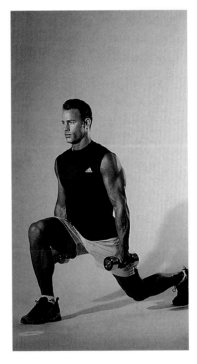

OVERHAND-GRIP
MACHINE ROW

1 Position yourself on the row machine with your chest against the pad, and grab the handles so that your palms face the floor.

2 Pull the handles back as far as you can. Pause, then slowly return to the starting position.

If you don't have access to this machine: Do a one-arm dumbbell row with your elbow out. Lean over a bench, resting your left knee and left hand on it. Hold a dumbbell in your right hand at arm's length, your right thumb facing your body. Pull the weight up until your elbow is bent 90 degrees, keeping your upper arm out away from your torso. Pause, then slowly lower the weight. Do all the repetitions with one arm (including the repetitions in the drop set, if you're doing the advanced routine), then repeat with the other.

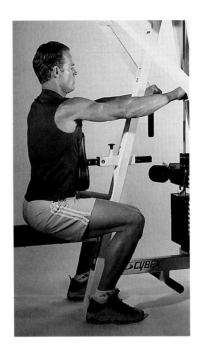 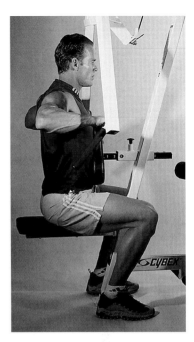

OWEN CRUNCH

1 Lie faceup on the floor with your hands behind your ears, your knees bent and together, and your toes pointing inward.

2 Raise your head and shoulders and crunch your rib cage toward your pelvis. Pause, then slowly return to the starting position.

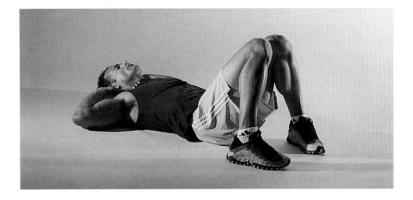

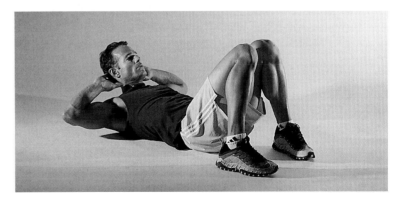

Men

SEX
6 NEW
TRICKS

LOS
10 LBS.
FAT

MUSCLE-U
YOUR CHE

**The Only Tv
Vitamins Y**

SEE YOUR
HEALTH F

THE BEE

THE MUSCLES
Cover Model Workout, **Phase 2**

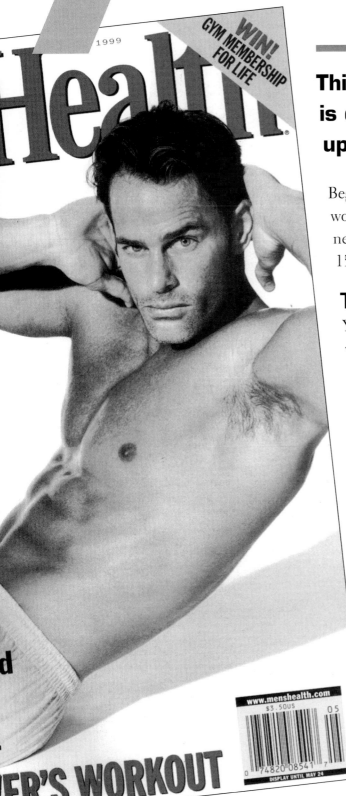

This 4-week program is designed to build serious upper-body muscle.

Beginners and advanced exercisers will do the same workouts this time—the only difference is that beginners will do more repetitions of each exercise (10 to 15) than advanced guys will (6 to 10).

The Goals

Your aim in Phase 2 is rapid, balanced muscle development, with some strength gains and continued improvement in muscle endurance. You'll work the muscles on the front of your body just as hard as the ones on the back.

The Routines

As in all four phases of the Cover Model Workout, you'll do three weight workouts each week. You'll do the core routine twice (preferably Monday and Friday) and the integrity routine once (Wednesday, most likely).

Core routine: The core routine in this chapter uses trisets—three different exercises for the same muscle group, performed without rest between them—to induce a level of muscular fatigue that produces rapid muscle gains. You'll do five trisets, one for each of your major upper-body muscle groups: chest, back, shoulders, biceps, and triceps.

Integrity routine: This month, the integrity routine hits your lower body with supersets—consecutive exercises for different muscle groups, performed without rest between them. The first exercise in each of the three supersets emphasizes one of the major lower-body muscle groups (gluteals and hamstrings, quadriceps, or calves), while the second hits your abdominals in slightly different ways.

Time

As in the first phase, you should finish all your workouts in well under an hour.

Warmup

Each workout, both beginner and advanced guys should do two warmup sets of the first exercise in the first triset or superset, then two warmup sets of the first exercise in the second triset or superset.

So before the core workout, do two warmup sets of the incline dumbbell bench press followed by two warmup sets of the lat pulldown. Then do your workout exactly as it's presented in the log. (You should be able to do the third, fourth, and fifth trisets—for your shoulders, biceps, and triceps—without any additional warmup.)

Before the integrity workout, do two warmup sets each of the dumbbell stepup and the dumbbell lunge, then proceed with your workout.

Speed

As in Phase 1, you want to perform repetitions deliberately (take 2 seconds to raise the weight, pause, take 3 or 4 seconds to lower the weight, pause). But by the time you get to the third exercise in each triset—particularly when you're at the end of your workout, working your biceps and triceps—you won't be doing anything deliberately. I still want you to try to move the weights slowly, however, even though I know you won't be able to. That's because I want you to stay in control of the weights at all times, no matter how tired you are. Controlled lifting not only minimizes the potential for injury but also builds the qualities I discussed in this book's opening chapters: persistence, discipline, and control over your destiny.

Rest between Trisets and Supersets

Take up to 2 minutes of rest between trisets in the core program, but try to keep it to 30 seconds or less between supersets in the integrity routine. As I noted in Phase 1, you may not be able to pull this off, especially if you exercise at home and are unable to change the weights that quickly in preparation for the next exercise. In that case, just move as fast as you can between exercises.

Cardiovascular Routine

I'll give detailed instructions after each weight routine.

Beginner Routine

Exercise	Reps	Week 1 Weight/Reps	Week 1 Weight/Reps	Week 2 Weight/Reps	Week 2 Weight/Reps	Week 3 Weight/Reps	Week 3 Weight/Reps	Week 4 Weight/Reps	Week 4 Weight/Reps
TRISET 1									
Incline dumbbell bench press	10–15								
Dumbbell bench press	10–15								
Decline dumbbell bench press	10–15								
Rest (up to 2 min)									
TRISET 2									
Lat pulldown	10–15								
Overhand-grip machine row	10–15								
Neutral-grip machine row	10–15								
Rest (up to 2 min)									
TRISET 3									
Dumbbell shoulder press	10–15								
Front-raise pullover	10–15								
Reverse fly	10–15								
Rest (up to 2 min)									
TRISET 4									
Reverse-grip biceps curl	10–15								
Biceps curl	10–15								
Hammer curl	10–15								
Rest (up to 2 min)									
TRISET 5									
Reverse wide-grip triceps pushdown	10–15								
Rope triceps pushdown	10–15								
Wide-grip triceps pushdown	10–15								

INTEGRITY WORKOUT: WEDNESDAYS

Exercise	Reps	Week 1	Week 2	Week 3	Week 4
		Weight/Reps	Weight/Reps	Weight/Reps	Weight/Reps
SUPERSET 1					
Dumbbell stepup	10–15				
Swiss-ball reverse crunch	10–15				
Rest (up to 30 sec)					
SUPERSET 2					
Dumbbell lunge	10–15				
Side jackknife	10–15				
Rest (up to 30 sec)					
SUPERSET 3					
Standing calf raise	10–15				
Swiss-ball crunch	10–15				

*"Maximum fitness—
and the health
that goes with it—
is its own reward."*

Cardiovascular-Training Workout

If you haven't done any cardiovascular exercise in the past 6 months, try the beginner routine in Phase 1 (see page 87).

If you already did that routine, you're ready to try the Phase-1 advanced cardio workout. It's a 20-minute, high-intensity interval routine that will prepare you for the more difficult interval routines in the later phases. And since high-intensity training stimulates your body to keep burning calories even after you finish exercising, you'll increase your metabolism after just one workout.

Perform each sprint described at right on a treadmill or an exercise bike at the prescribed percentage of your highest possible effort (see "Rating Your Cardio Effort" on page 88 to determine each percentage). Then, slow to an active rest at a lower intensity—a light jog, for instance.

Warm up for 5 minutes, gradually increasing your intensity to about 50 percent of full effort.

→ Sprint for 30 seconds at 85 percent of full effort.
→ Take an active rest for 2 minutes at 45 percent of full effort.
→ Sprint for 20 seconds at 90 percent of full effort.
→ Take an active rest for 2 minutes at 45 percent of full effort.
→ Sprint for 10 seconds at 100 percent (full sprint).
→ Take an active rest for 2 minutes at 45 percent of full effort.
→ Sprint for 20 seconds at 90 percent of full effort.
→ Take an active rest for 2 minutes at 45 percent of full effort.
→ Sprint for 30 seconds at 85 percent of full effort.
→ Cool down for 5 minutes.

"Sprinting is the quintessential Cover Model Workout exercise."

Advanced Routine

CORE WORKOUT: MONDAYS AND FRIDAYS

Exercise	Reps	Week 1 Weight/Reps	Week 1 Weight/Reps	Week 2 Weight/Reps	Week 2 Weight/Reps	Week 3 Weight/Reps	Week 3 Weight/Reps	Week 4 Weight/Reps	Week 4 Weight/Reps
TRISET 1									
Incline dumbbell bench press	6–10								
Dumbbell bench press	6–10								
Decline dumbbell bench press	6–10								
Rest (up to 2 min)									
TRISET 2									
Lat pulldown	6–10								
Overhand-grip machine row	6–10								
Neutral-grip machine row	6–10								
Rest (up to 2 min)									
TRISET 3									
Dumbbell shoulder press	6–10								
Front-raise pullover	6–10								
Reverse fly	6–10								
Rest (up to 2 min)									
TRISET 4									
Reverse-grip biceps curl	6–10								
Biceps curl	6–10								
Hammer curl	6–10								
Rest (up to 2 min)									
TRISET 5									
Reverse wide-grip triceps pushdown	6–10								
Rope triceps pushdown	6–10								
Wide-grip triceps pushdown	6–10								

INTEGRITY WORKOUT: WEDNESDAYS

Exercise	Reps	Week 1	Week 2	Week 3	Week 4
		Weight/Reps	Weight/Reps	Weight/Reps	Weight/Reps
SUPERSET 1					
Dumbbell stepup	6–10				
Swiss-ball reverse crunch	6–10				
Rest (up to 30 sec)					
SUPERSET 2					
Dumbbell lunge	6–10				
Side jackknife	6–10				
Rest (up to 30 sec)					
SUPERSET 3					
Standing calf raise	6–10				
Swiss-ball crunch	6–10				

"Permanent change
comes only with persistence.
The payoff is worth it."

Cardiovascular-Training Workout

If you've been doing cardiovascular exercise consistently for the past 6 months, try this 20-minute, high-intensity interval routine. It'll prepare you for the more difficult interval routines in the next three phases. And since high-intensity training stimulates your body to keep burning calories even after you finish exercising, you'll increase your metabolism after just one workout.

Perform each sprint described at right on a treadmill or an exercise bike at the prescribed percentage of your highest possible effort (see "Rating Your Cardio Effort" on page 88 to determine each percentage). Then, slow to an active rest at a lower intensity—a light jog, for instance.

Warm up for 5 minutes, gradually increasing your intensity to about 50 percent of full effort.

→ Sprint for 30 seconds at 85 percent of full effort.
→ Take an active rest for 2 minutes at 45 percent of full effort.
→ Sprint for 20 seconds at 90 percent of full effort.
→ Take an active rest for 2 minutes at 45 percent of full effort.
→ Sprint for 10 seconds at 100 percent (full sprint).
→ Take an active rest for 2 minutes at 45 percent of full effort.
→ Sprint for 20 seconds at 90 percent of full effort.
→ Take an active rest for 2 minutes at 45 percent of full effort.
→ Sprint for 30 seconds at 85 percent of full effort.
→ Cool down for 5 minutes.

The Exercises

INCLINE DUMBBELL BENCH PRESS

1 Adjust a bench to a 10- to 30-degree incline. Grab a pair of dumbbells and sit on the bench. Hold the dumbbells just outside your shoulders, with your arms bent and your palms facing forward.

2 Push the weights up and slightly inward so that when your arms are extended, the dumbbells are above your collarbones. Lower the weights back to your chest, and pause before repeating.

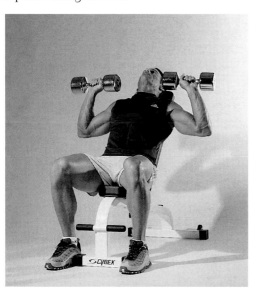

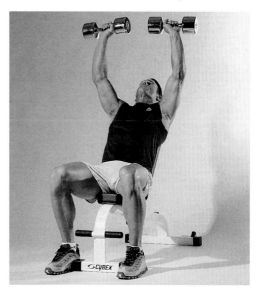

DUMBBELL BENCH PRESS

1 Grab a pair of dumbbells and lie faceup on a flat bench. Hold the dumbbells just outside your shoulders, with your arms bent and your palms facing your feet.

2 Push the weights up and slightly inward so that when your arms are extended, the dumbbells are above your collarbones. Lower the weights back to your chest, and pause before repeating.

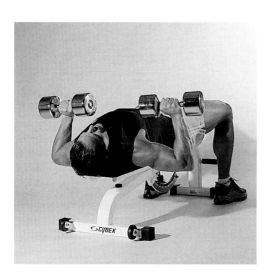

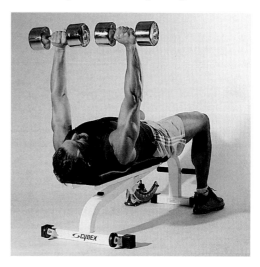

DECLINE DUMBBELL BENCH PRESS

1 Grab a pair of dumbbells and lie faceup on a decline bench with your feet under the leg supports. Hold the dumbbells just outside your shoulders, with your arms bent and your palms facing forward.

2 Push the weights straight up until your arms are extended. Lower the weights back to your chest, and pause before repeating.

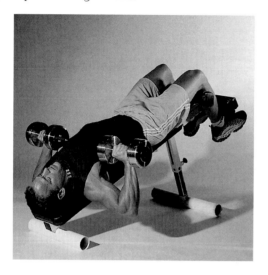 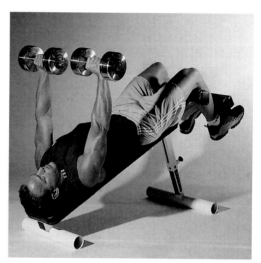

LAT PULLDOWN

1 Sit at a lat-pulldown station and grab the bar with a "false" overhand grip that's just beyond shoulder-width. A false grip means you place your thumb on top of the bar, alongside your index finger, rather than wrap it around the bar.

2 Pull the bar down to your chest. Pause, then slowly return to the starting position.

If you don't have access to this machine: Do a pullover with dumbbells. Lie faceup on a bench and hold the weights over your chest with your arms extended, your elbows slightly bent, and your palms facing your toes. The weights should be perpendicular to the floor. Keeping your back flat against the bench to elongate your lats, slowly lower the weights behind your head until your upper arms are parallel to the floor. Then pull the weights back to the starting position. Keep a slight bend in your elbows throughout.

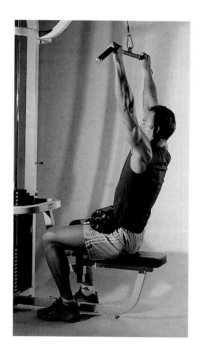 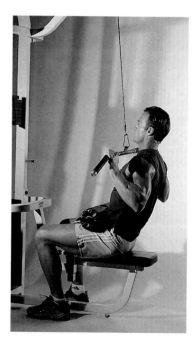

OVERHAND-GRIP MACHINE ROW

1 Position yourself on a row machine with your chest against the pad, and grab the handles so that your palms face the floor.

2 Pull the handles back as far as you can. Pause, then slowly return to the starting position.

If you don't have access to this machine: Do a one-arm dumbbell row with your elbow out. Lean over a bench, resting your left knee and left hand on it. Hold a dumbbell in your right hand at arm's length, your right thumb facing your body. Pull the weight up until your elbow is bent 90 degrees, keeping your upper arm out away from your torso. Pause, then slowly lower the weight. Do all the repetitions with one arm (including the repetitions in the drop set, if you're doing the advanced routine), then repeat with the other.

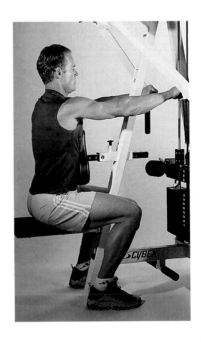
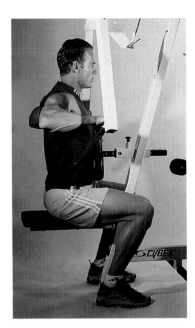

NEUTRAL-GRIP MACHINE ROW

1 Position yourself on a row machine with your chest against the pad, and grab the handles so that your palms face each other.

2 Pull the handles back as far as you can. Pause, then slowly return to the starting position.

If you don't have access to this machine: Do a one-arm dumbbell row with your palm facing in. Lean over a bench, resting your left knee and left hand on it. Hold a dumbbell in your right hand at arm's length, with your palm facing your body. Keeping your upper arm tucked against your torso, pull the weight up until your elbow is bent 90 degrees. Pause, then slowly lower the weight. Do all the repetitions with one arm (including the repetitions in the drop set, if you're doing the advanced routine), then repeat with the other.

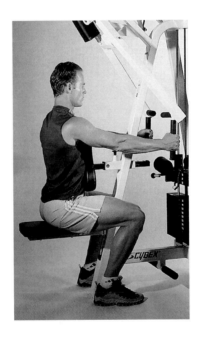
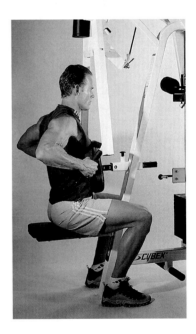

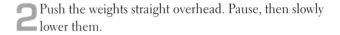

DUMBBELL SHOULDER PRESS

1 Grab a pair of dumbbells and sit holding them just outside your shoulders, with your arms bent and your palms facing each other.

2 Push the weights straight overhead. Pause, then slowly lower them.

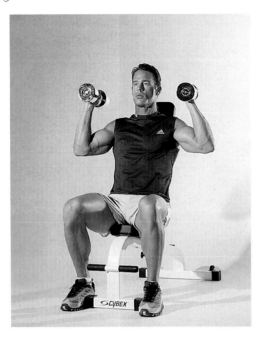
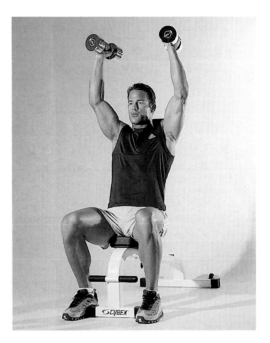

FRONT-RAISE PULLOVER

1 Grab a weight plate in both hands, and hold it with bent arms in front of your hips and midsection. Stagger your feet so your left foot is in front of you.

2 Without changing the bend in your elbows, raise your arms until your forearms are nearly perpendicular to the floor. Contract your abdominal muscles as you lift the weight. Pause, then lower to the starting position.

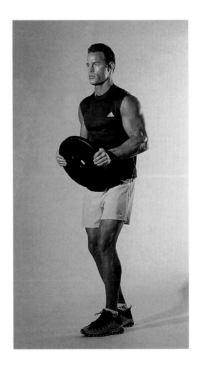
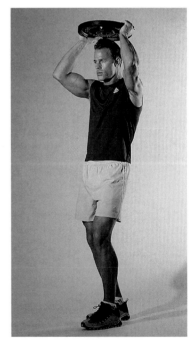

REVERSE FLY

1 Grab a pair of dumbbells and sit at the end of a bench. Lean forward at the waist as far as you can, keeping your back flat and your elbows slightly bent. Let the dumbbells hang at arm's length, with your thumbs turned toward each other.

2 Slowly raise the weights as high as you can without changing the angle of your elbows. Pause, then lower to the starting position.

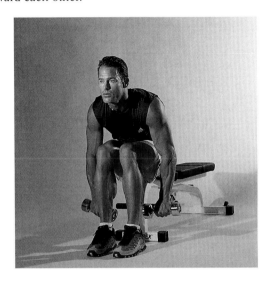

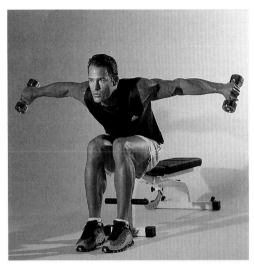

REVERSE-GRIP BICEPS CURL

1 Grab an EZ-curl barbell (that's the bar shaped like a **W** in the middle) with an overhand, shoulder-width grip (in other words, grab the outer edges of the **W**). Stand with your feet staggered so your left foot is in front of you; keep your knees slightly bent and your back straight. Hold the bar at arm's length, in front of your thighs.

2 Curl the bar upward as high as you can without moving your upper arms—they should stay tucked against your sides. Pause, then slowly return to the starting position.

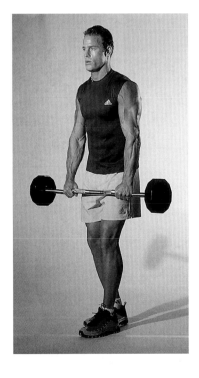

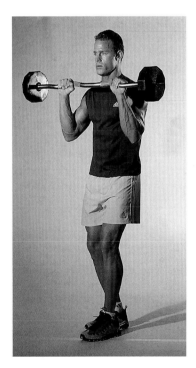

BICEPS CURL

1 Grab an EZ-curl bar with an underhand, shoulder-width grip. Stand with your feet staggered so your left foot is in front of you; keep your knees slightly bent and your back straight. Hold the bar at arm's length, in front of your thighs. Keep your upper arms tucked against your sides.

2 Curl the bar as high as you can without letting your upper arms move forward. Pause, then slowly return to the starting position.

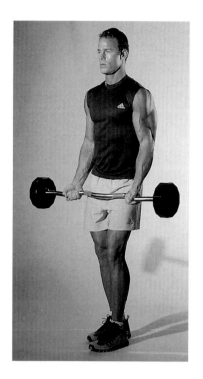 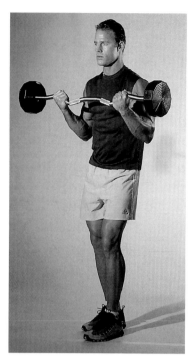

HAMMER CURL

1 Grab a pair of dumbbells and stand with your feet staggered so your left foot is in front of you. Let your arms hang straight down from your shoulders, and turn your hands so your palms face each other.

2 Moving only from the elbows, curl the weights up as high as you can. Pause, then slowly lower them to the starting position.

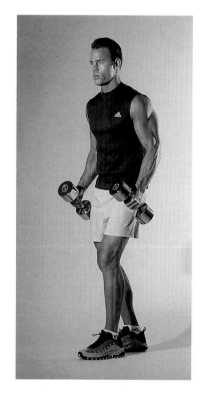 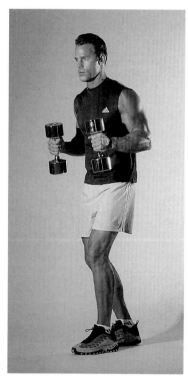

REVERSE WIDE-GRIP TRICEPS PUSHDOWN

1 Attach a straight bar to the high pulley of a cable station. Grab the bar with an underhand, shoulder-width grip and pull it down until your elbows are bent 90 degrees. Stand straight, with your upper arms tucked against your sides. Keep your feet hip-width apart and your knees slightly bent.

2 Push the handle down until your arms are straight, keeping the rest of your body in the starting position. Pause, then slowly allow the handle to rise until your elbows are bent 90 degrees.

If you don't have access to this machine: Do a reverse-grip "skull-crusher." Lie faceup on a flat bench, holding an EZ-curl bar at arm's length over your chin with a reverse grip (palms facing your head). Without moving your upper arms, bend your elbows to slowly lower the bar until it's just at your forehead or just behind it. Pause, then straighten your elbows.

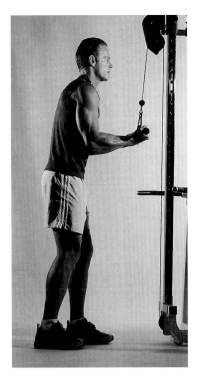 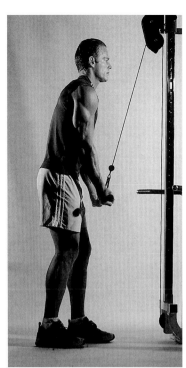

ROPE TRICEPS PUSHDOWN

1 Attach a rope handle to the high pulley of a cable station and grab it so your palms face each other. Start with your elbows bent 90 degrees and your upper arms against your sides.

2 Straighten your arms, allowing your hands to pull the rope ends outward at the bottom. Pause, then slowly return to the starting position.

If you don't have access to this machine: Do a seated dumbbell triceps extension. Grab a pair of dumbbells and sit on a bench or chair. Hold the dumbbells overhead with straight arms. Bend at the elbows to slowly lower the weights behind and to the sides of your head. Hold your upper arms in the same position. Pause, then push up to the starting position.

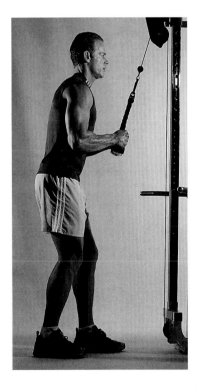 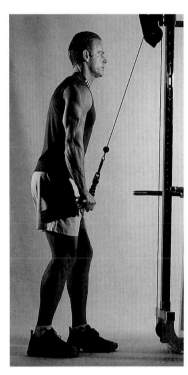

WIDE-GRIP TRICEPS PUSHDOWN

1 Attach a straight bar to the high pulley of a cable station. Grab the bar with an overhand, shoulder-width grip and pull it down until your elbows are bent 90 degrees. Stand straight, with your upper arms tucked against your sides. Keep your feet hip-width apart and your knees slightly bent.

2 Push the bar down until your arms are straight, keeping the rest of your body in the starting position. It's crucial to keep your upper arms against your sides. Pause, then slowly allow the bar to rise until your elbows are again bent 90 degrees.

If you don't have access to this machine: Do a "skullcrusher." Lie faceup on a flat bench, holding an EZ-curl bar at arm's length over your chin with your palms facing your feet. Without moving your upper arms, bend your elbows to slowly lower the bar until it's just at your forehead or just behind it. Pause, then straighten your elbows.

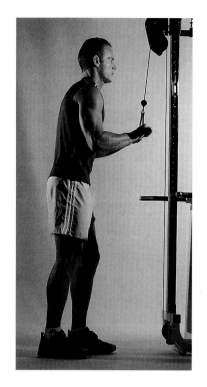
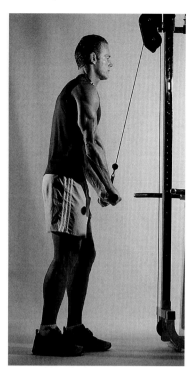

DUMBBELL STEPUP

1 Grab a pair of dumbbells and stand facing a step or bench that's 6 to 12 inches off the floor.

2 Lift your nondominant foot (your left if you're right-handed) and place it firmly on the bench.

Push down with that heel, and step up onto the bench so you're standing on it with both feet. Step down with your dominant foot first, then with your nondominant. Finish the set with your nondominant leg, then do the same number of repetitions starting with your other foot.

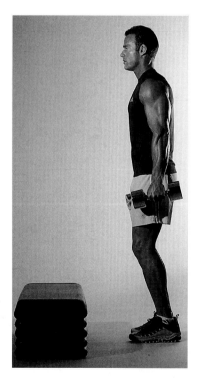
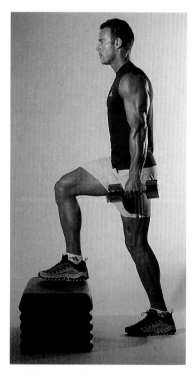

SWISS-BALL REVERSE CRUNCH

1 Lie on a slant board with your hips lower than your head. Grab the bar behind your head for support. Bend your hips and knees at 90-degree angles and hold a small Swiss ball between your hamstrings and your calves. Start with your butt flat against the board.

2 Pull your hips up and in toward your rib cage, as if emptying a bucket of water that was resting on your pelvis. Curl them as high as you can without lifting your shoulders off the board, and keep your hips and knees at 90-degree angles. Pause, then slowly return to the starting position. If this exercise is too difficult, perform it on the floor or without the Swiss ball.

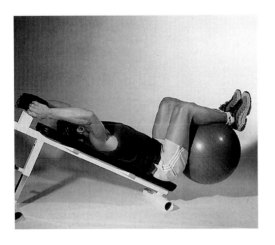
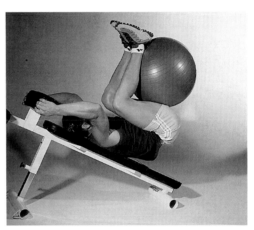

DUMBBELL LUNGE

1 Grab a pair of dumbbells and hold them at your sides. Stand with your feet hip-width apart.

2 Step forward with your nondominant leg (your left if you're right-handed), and lower your body until your front knee is bent 90 degrees and your rear knee nearly touches the floor. Your front lower leg should be perpendicular to the floor, and your torso should remain upright. Push yourself back up to the starting position as quickly as you can, and repeat with your dominant leg. That's 1 repetition.

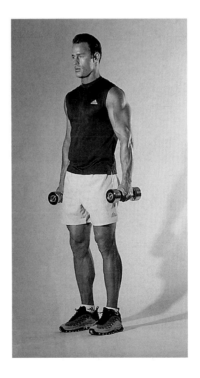
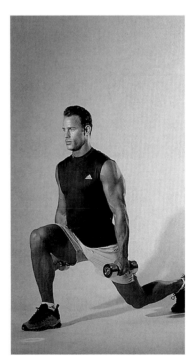

SIDE JACKKNIFE

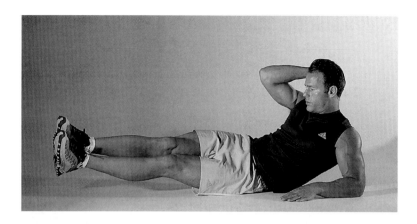

1 Lie on your left hip, with your legs nearly straight and slightly raised off the floor. Also raise your torso off the floor, with your left forearm on the floor for balance. Hold your other hand behind your right ear, with your elbow pointed toward your feet.

2 Lift your legs toward your torso, while keeping your torso stationary. Pause to feel the contraction on the right side of your waist. Then slowly lower your legs and repeat. Finish the set on that side, then lie on your right hip and do the same number of repetitions.

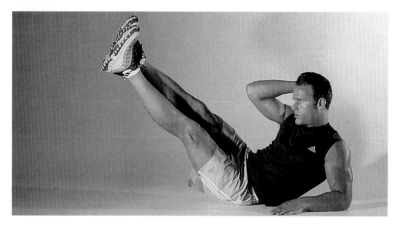

STANDING CALF RAISE

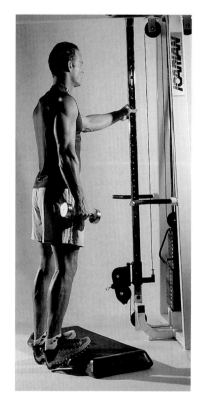
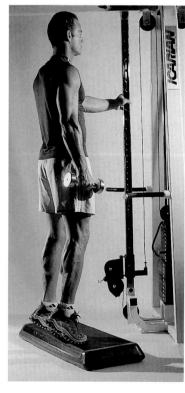

1 Grab a dumbbell in one hand and stand on the balls of your feet on a step or block. Steady yourself by using your other hand to hold on to a stable object—a weight stack or wall, for instance. Lower your heels as far as you can.

2 Rise up on your toes as high as you can. Pause, then slowly lower your heels.

SWISS-BALL CRUNCH

1 Lie faceup on a Swiss ball, with your hands behind your ears.

2 Raise your head and shoulders, and crunch your rib cage toward your pelvis. Pause, then slowly return to the starting position.

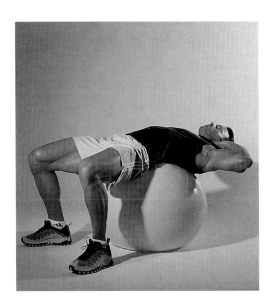

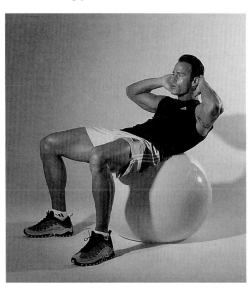

8 THE STRENGTH

Cover Model Workout, **Phase 3**

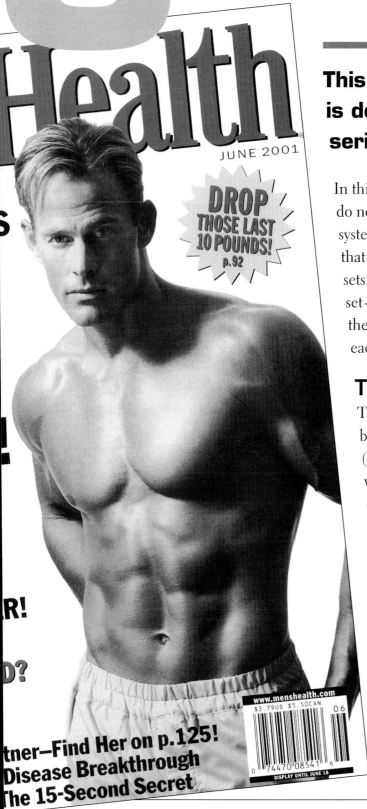

Health

JUNE 2001

DROP THOSE LAST 10 POUNDS! p.92

R!

D?

www.menshealth.com
$3.79US $5.50CAN
06

tner—Find Her on p.125!
Disease Breakthrough
The 15-Second Secret

0 74470 08541 6
DISPLAY UNTIL JUNE 18

This 4-week program is designed to build serious total-body strength.

In this phase, beginners and advanced exercisers will do not only the same workout but also the same system of sets and repetitions. The one difference is that beginners will probably choose to do fewer sets—perhaps the two warmup sets and one work set—while advanced guys will probably want to do the maximum: two warmups and three work sets of each exercise.

The Goals

The core workout builds pure upper- and lower-body strength, with some increases in muscle mass (especially for more advanced lifters). The integrity workout focuses on building muscle mass and endurance in the shoulders and elbows, joints that can take a beating in a strength program.

The Routines

As in all four phases of the Cover Model Workout, do three weight workouts each week. Do the core routine twice (preferably Monday and Friday) and the integrity routine once (Wednesday, most likely).

Core routine: The core routine in this chapter includes five exercises and gives you the option of doing five sets of each: two warmups and one to three work sets. It's up to you how many of the work sets you do on each exercise. You may start with one the first week, two the second week, and three the third and fourth weeks. Or you could do three from the first week on. Use the same amount of weight for each work set.

Whatever you do, it's crucial that you try to increase the amount of weight you use each week. Increase the weight as soon as you can do eight repetitions in all work sets with a given weight.

Integrity routine: This month, the integrity routine hits your smaller upper-body muscles—deltoids, biceps, triceps—with drop sets. You'll do one set of up to 15 repetitions, then drop the weight about 20 percent and immediately do another set of up to 10 reps.

Time

As in the previous phases, you should finish all your workouts in well under an hour.

Warmup

The warmup sets in the core workout are mandatory for both beginners and advanced guys. Use about 50 percent of your work-set weight in the first warmup set, and about 75 percent in the second.

Before the integrity workout, warmup sets aren't necessary as long as you do a general warmup as described in Phase 1: calisthenics or 5 minutes on a treadmill or exercise bike.

Speed

In both the core and integrity workouts, you should let your body tell you how fast to lift the weights. You don't want to lift as deliberately as you did in previous phases, since that means using lighter weights. And lighter weights aren't the idea. Still, you don't want to fling the weights around carelessly. You need to control the weights on all your lifts, and never allow your form to suffer for the sake of getting an extra repetition or two. Ideally, you'll take about 1 second to lift the weight and 2 seconds to lower it.

In the integrity workout, you aren't lifting particularly heavy weights—not if you're going to get 15 reps in the first set and 10 in the second—but you still don't want to lift at an artificially slow speed. Ideally, you'll take 2 seconds to raise the weight and 1 to lower it.

Rest between Sets and Drop Sets

Take at least a minute, and as much as 3 minutes, between sets in the core routine. (You don't have to take that much time between warmup sets, however.) The more time you rest between sets, the more weight you'll be able to lift, and that's the whole point of the program.

In the integrity routine, you don't need to take a lot of time between exercises. It may take you a minute to set up for the next exercise, and that's plenty of rest. Obviously, you don't want to rest at all between sets in a drop set. Do the first, then begin the second as soon as you can lower the weight 20 percent.

Cardiovascular Routine

I'll give detailed instructions after the weight routine, on page 124.

Beginner and Advanced Routine

CORE WORKOUT: MONDAYS AND FRIDAYS

Exercise	Reps	Week 1 Weight/Reps	Week 1 Weight/Reps	Week 2 Weight/Reps	Week 2 Weight/Reps	Week 3 Weight/Reps	Week 3 Weight/Reps	Week 4 Weight/Reps	Week 4 Weight/Reps
Deep squat									
Warmup set 1 ($1/2$ of work-set weight)	6								
Warmup set 2 ($3/4$ of work-set weight)	6								
Work set 1	5–8								
Rest (1–3 min)									
Work set 2	5–8								
Rest (1–3 min)									
Work set 3	5–8								
Lat pulldown (or pullup*)									
Warmup set 1 ($1/2$ of work-set weight)	6								
Warmup set 2 ($3/4$ of work-set weight)	6								
Work set 1	5–8								
Rest (1–3 min)									
Work set 2	5–8								
Rest (1–3 min)									
Work set 3	5–8								
Decline dumbbell bench press									
Warmup set 1 ($1/2$ of work-set weight)	6								
Warmup set 2 ($3/4$ of work-set weight)	6								
Work set 1	5–8								
Rest (1–3 min)									

* If you can do more than 8 pullups per set, do weighted pullups for your work sets, using a belt that allows you to hang a dumbbell or weight plate from your waist. For your warmups, you can use your body weight, or do lat pulldowns with a percentage of your combined body weight and the extra weight you plan to hang from the belt.

CORE WORKOUT: MONDAYS AND FRIDAYS

Exercise	Reps	Week 1	Week 1	Week 2	Week 2	Week 3	Week 3	Week 4	Week 4
		Weight/Reps	Weight/Reps	Weight/Reps	Weight/Reps	Weight/Reps	Weight/Reps	Weight/Reps	Weight/Reps
Decline dumbbell bench press									
Work set 2	5–8								
Rest (1–3 min)									
Work set 3	5–8								
Romanian deadlift									
Warmup set 1 ($^1/_2$ of work-set weight)	6								
Warmup set 2 ($^3/_4$ of work-set weight)	6								
Work set 1	5–8								
Rest (1–3 min)									
Work set 2	5–8								
Rest (1–3 min)									
Work set 3	5–8								
Weighted Swiss-ball crunch									
Warmup set 1 ($^1/_2$ of work-set weight)	6								
Warmup set 2 ($^3/_4$ of work-set weight)	6								
Work set 1	5–8								
Rest (1–3 min)									
Work set 2	5–8								
Rest (1–3 min)									
Work set 3	5–8								

INTEGRITY WORKOUT: WEDNESDAYS

Exercise	Reps	Week 1	Week 2	Week 3	Week 4
		Weight/Reps	Weight/Reps	Weight/Reps	Weight/Reps
Curl-and-press					
Set 1	15				
Set 2 (drop)	10				
Lateral raise					
Set 1	15				
Set 2 (drop)	10				
90-degree lateral raise					
Set 1	15				
Set 2 (drop)	10				
Reverse-grip dumbbell shoulder press					
Set 1	15				
Set 2 (drop)	10				
Single-arm thumb-down shoulder raise					
Set 1	15				
Set 2 (drop)	10				
Single-arm reverse fly					
Set 1	15				
Set 2 (drop)	10				
Lying triceps kickback					
Set 1	15				
Set 2 (drop)	10				

Cardiovascular-Training Workout

You can do your cardiovascular training immediately after your weight work or on separate days. If you haven't done any aerobic work in the past 6 months, or if you are more than 15 pounds overweight, start out by walking or riding a bike (or stationary cycle) for 10 to 15 minutes. If you use a treadmill, set it on a slight incline—2 to 5 degrees; otherwise, it's easier than walking outdoors. The intensity doesn't matter, especially in the first week. You should always finish your cardiovascular exercise feeling as if you could've done more. Try to go about 10 percent longer each week. Or go a little harder in the same amount of time—increase the incline or speed of the treadmill, for example. Once you've worked up to 20 to 30 minutes of continuous exercise, start with the advanced cardiovascular routines described in Phases 1 and 2 (see pages 91 and 106).

If you've already done the Phase-1 and -2 advanced cardio workouts, try this high-intensity interval routine. It's designed to maximize the amount of time it takes until your body is fatigued. So you'll be able to exercise harder and longer. Plus, it increases the amount of time you are actually performing high-intensity exercise, allowing you to burn more fat during—and after—your workout.

Perform a 30-second sprint on a track, treadmill, or exercise bike, at your highest possible effort. Slow into an active rest at a lower intensity—a light jog or walk—for 150 seconds. Your active rest should be slow enough that your breathing returns to normal by the end of 90 seconds.

Warm up for 5 minutes, gradually increasing your intensity to about 50 percent of full effort.

→ Week 1: 5 sprints
→ Week 2: 6 sprints
→ Week 3: 7 sprints
→ Week 4: 8 sprints
→ Cool down for 5 minutes.

"The resistance programs in the Cover Model Workout emphasize muscle performance over sheer muscle size."

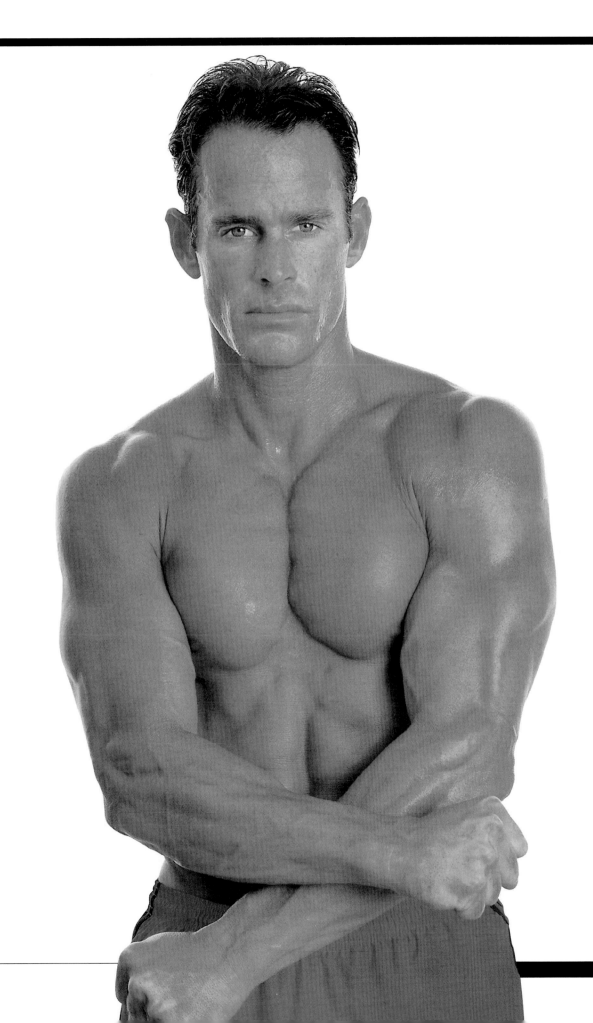

The Exercises

DEEP SQUAT

1 Set a barbell on a squat rack and step under it so the bar rests across your upper back. Pull your shoulders back as you grab the bar with an overhand grip. The bar should sit comfortably on your upper trapezius muscles. Lift the bar off the rack and step back. Set your feet shoulder-width apart; keep your knees slightly bent, your back straight, and your eyes focused straight ahead.

2 Slowly lower your body as if you were sitting back into a chair, keeping your back in its natural alignment and your lower legs nearly perpendicular to the floor. When you have squatted as far down as possible, pause before returning to the starting position.

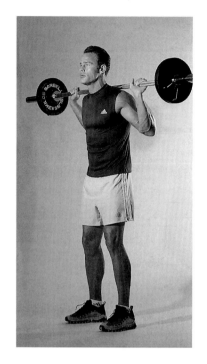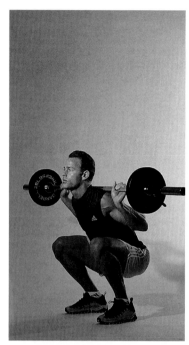

LAT PULLDOWN

1 Sit at a lat-pulldown station and grab the bar with a "false" overhand grip that's just beyond shoulder-width. A false grip means you place your thumb on top of the bar, alongside your index finger, rather than wrap it around the bar.

2 Pull the bar down to your chest. Pause, then slowly return to the starting position.

If you don't have access to this machine: Do a pullover with dumbbells. Lie faceup on a bench and hold the weights over your chest with your arms extended, your elbows slightly bent, and your palms facing your toes. The weights should be perpendicular to the floor. Keeping your back flat against the bench to elongate your lats, slowly lower the weights behind your head until your upper arms are parallel to the floor. Keep a slight bend in your elbows throughout. Then pull back to the starting position.

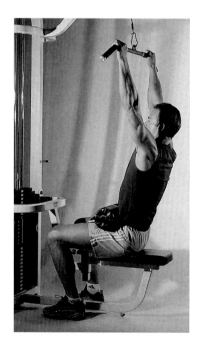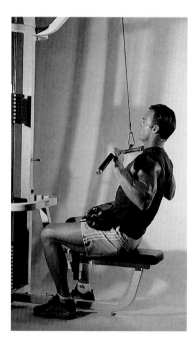

PULLUP

1 Grab a pullup bar with an overhand grip, your hands just outside shoulder-width. Hang at arm's length with your knees bent and your feet crossed behind you.

2 Pull yourself up until your chin passes the bar. Pause, then slowly lower yourself.

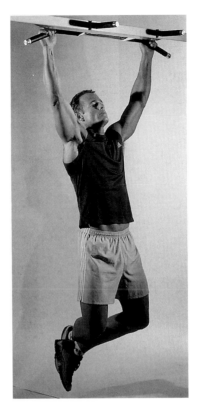
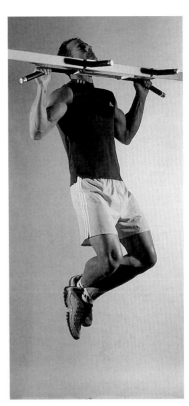

DECLINE DUMBBELL BENCH PRESS

1 Grab a pair of dumbbells and lie faceup on a decline bench with your feet under the leg supports. Hold the dumbbells just outside your shoulders, with your arms bent and your palms facing forward.

2 Push the weights straight up until your arms are extended. Lower the weights back to your chest, and pause before repeating.

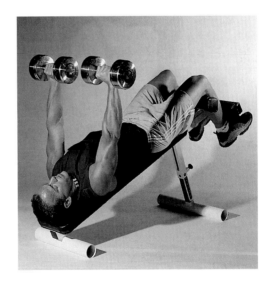

ROMANIAN DEADLIFT

1 Grab a barbell with an overhand grip that's just beyond shoulder-width. Stand holding the bar at arm's length, resting it on the fronts of your thighs. Keep your feet shoulder-width apart, your knees slightly bent, and your eyes focused straight ahead. Pull your shoulders back.

2 Slowly bend at the waist as you lower the bar to just below your knees. Don't change the angle of your knees. Keep your head and chest up and your lower back arched. Lift your torso back to the starting position, keeping the bar as close to your body as possible.

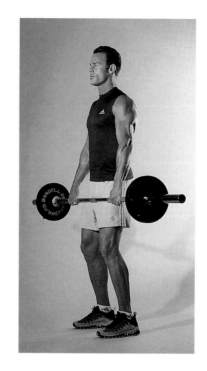 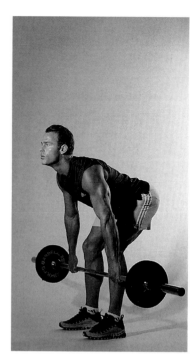

WEIGHTED SWISS-BALL CRUNCH

1 Lie faceup on a Swiss ball, with your hands under your chin, holding a weight plate or dumbbell.

2 Raise your head and shoulders and crunch your rib cage toward your pelvis. Pause, then slowly return to the starting position.

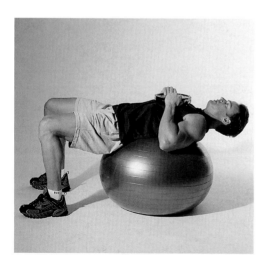 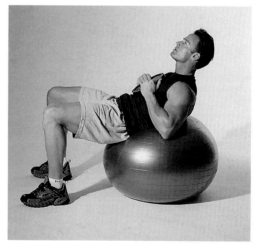

CURL-AND-PRESS

1 Grab a pair of dumbbells and sit upright on a bench. Let your arms hang straight down from your shoulders, and turn your palms forward.

2 Curl the weights upward as high as you can without moving your upper arms—they should stay tucked against your sides.

3 Then, turn your palms so they face away from you, and press the weights over your head. Reverse the sequence to lower the weights back down to the starting position.

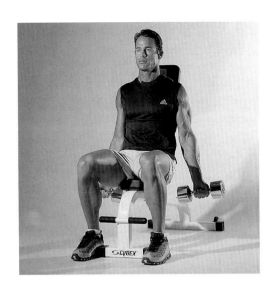

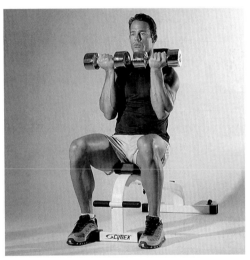

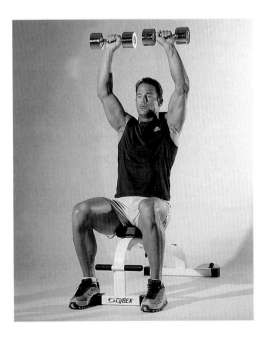

LATERAL RAISE

1 Grab a pair of dumbbells and sit holding them at arm's length with your palms turned toward each other. Bend your elbows slightly.

2 Without changing the bend in your elbows, raise your arms out to the sides until they're parallel to the floor. Pause, then lower them back to the starting position.

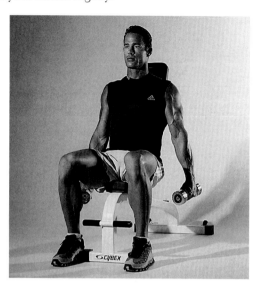 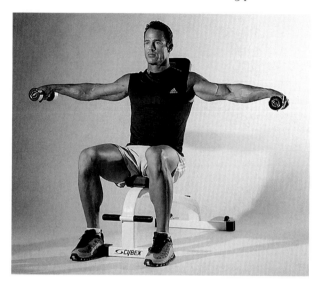

90-DEGREE LATERAL RAISE

1 Grab a pair of dumbbells and sit holding them in front of you with your elbows bent 90 degrees and your palms turned toward each other.

2 Without changing the bend in your elbows, raise your arms out to the sides until they are parallel to the floor. Pause, then lower them to the starting position.

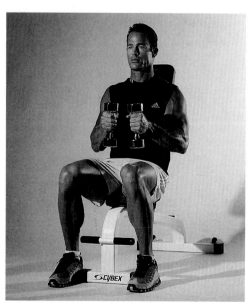 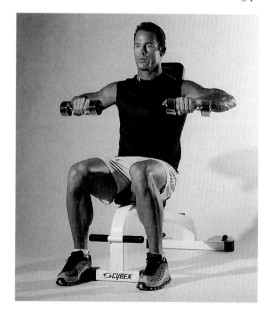

REVERSE-GRIP DUMBBELL SHOULDER PRESS

1 Grab a pair of dumbbells and sit holding them just in front of your shoulders, with your arms bent and your palms facing your shoulders.

2 Push the weights overhead, turning your palms so they face away from you in the top positon. Pause, then slowly lower the weights, twisting them back to the starting position.

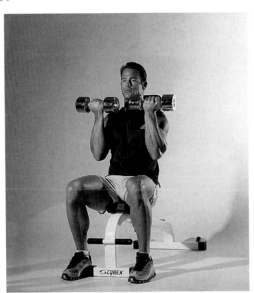 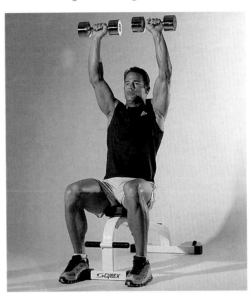

SINGLE-ARM THUMB-DOWN SHOULDER RAISE

1 Grab a dumbbell with your nondominant hand (your left if you're right-handed). Lie on your dominant side on a bench, placing your free hand on the floor to brace yourself. Extend your working arm, with your thumb pointing down and your elbow slightly bent, and raise it until it's just above parallel to the floor.

2 Without changing the bend in your elbow, slowly lower the weight until your arm is down toward the floor. Pause, then raise to the starting position. Finish the set with that arm, then do the same number of reps with your dominant arm.

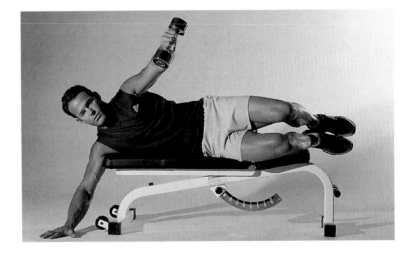

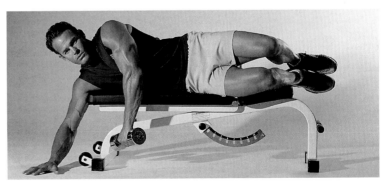

SINGLE-ARM REVERSE FLY

1 Grab a dumbbell with your nondominant hand (your left if you're right-handed). Lie on your dominant side on a bench, placing that elbow on the bench to brace yourself. Extend your working arm, with your palm facing down and your elbow slightly bent, and raise it to a 45-degree angle with the floor.

2 Slowly lower the weight behind your body until your working elbow starts to bend. Pause, then return to the starting position. Finish the set with that arm, then do the same number of reps with your dominant arm.

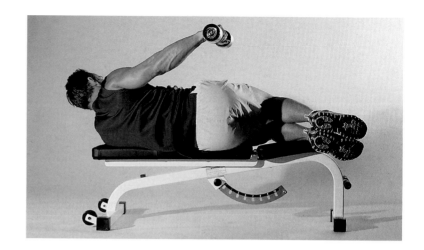

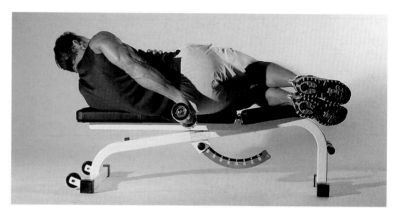

LYING TRICEPS KICKBACK

1 Grab a pair of dumbbells and lie facedown on a bench. Raise your upper arms so that they are parallel to the floor, and bend your elbows 90 degrees.

2 Straighten your arms by raising your forearms while keeping your upper arms in the same position. Pause, then lower to the starting position.

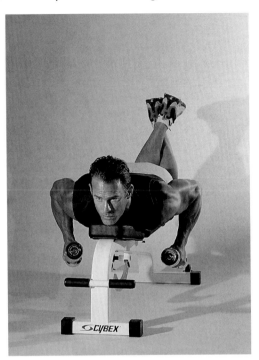
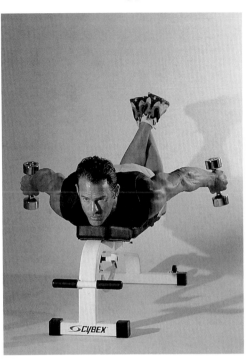

Men

Strong B
Tough M

Look Great!
44 Male Style
Secrets

BUILD BICEPS
THAT SHOW

LAST LONGER
IN BED

BEST
WINTER
WORKOUT

ULTIMATE
VITAMINS

THE BODY

Cover Model Workout, **Phase 4**

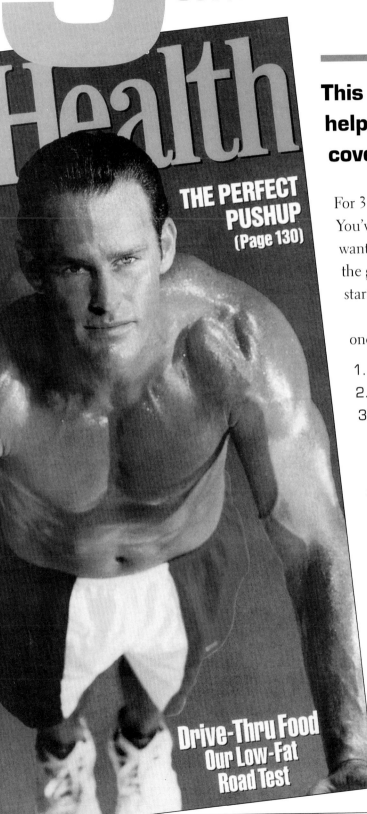

THE PERFECT PUSHUP
(Page 130)

Drive-Thru Food
Our Low-Fat
Road Test

This 3-week program helps you hone your cover model look.

For 3 months, you've done what I've told you to do: You've built endurance, muscle, and strength. Now, I want you to decide which you need most to achieve the goals you had when you bought this book and started this program.

Beginner and advanced guys alike should choose one of the following three core workouts.

1. Maximum fat loss
2. Maximum strength
3. Maximum muscle

A few words about each:

The fat-loss workout is simple but by no means easy. You do just three exercises, but with aerobic intervals in between. You burn calories by the bucket. It's one of the most metabolically demanding workouts you'll ever encounter, and it was designed in the spirit of my favorite workout: the one in which I run the Santa Monica Stairs, then walk down and do a set of pullups before running up again.

The strength workout doubles as a serious muscle-building workout for the most advanced lifters. It also includes just three exercises, but those exercises hit your body's biggest muscles. If you've been lifting consistently for a number of years—say, more than 3 years—your body probably responds best to this type of routine, using heavy weights and low repetitions.

The muscle workout is for lean guys who've been training consistently for up to 3 years. The principles are the same as those in the strength workout, except there are four exercises and they aren't as demanding, so you don't rest as much between sets.

The Goals

Hmm . . . a fat-loss workout, a strength workout, and a muscle workout. Nope, can't think of any goals you'd associate with the three core programs in this phase.

The Phase-4 integrity workout is the same for everyone. You'll develop the muscles surrounding your knee, shoulder, and elbow joints, with some abdominal sets to help support your lower back.

The Routines

Just as in the previous three phases of the Cover Model Workout, you'll do three weight workouts each week. Twice a week (preferable Monday and Friday), you'll do whichever core routine is applicable to your goal. Once weekly (probably Wednesday), you'll do the integrity routine.

CORE ROUTINE

Fat-loss workout: You'll perform each of the three exercises four times. After doing the first exercise, the squat-and-press, do a 2-minute cardio interval. The best exercise for this interval is jumping rope, but it's also the toughest. So do

"You can overcome any obstacle between you and an aesthetically appealing, healthy physique."

whatever you can. If you can jump rope, great. If not, run or walk on a treadmill, or ride an exercise bike for 2 minutes. If you can't jump rope and don't have access to cardio machines, do jumping jacks, walk up and down steps, or march in place.

Then do the bent-over row and dumbbell bench press without a break in between. After the bench press, do a 3-minute cardio interval.

Then immediately repeat the whole circuit three times. The object is to go for as long as you can without resting.

Strength workout: Do a set of deadlifts (the first exercise in the workout). Rest for 2 minutes. Do a set of dumbbell bench presses. Without resting after the bench presses, do a set of squats. Then rest for 3 minutes. Repeat until you've done the circuit five times. You'll feel that you're spending most of your workout waiting to begin the next set, rather than actually lifting (which is accurate), but these long rest periods will let you handle heavier weights when you do lift. That means more strength, which means more muscle.

Muscle workout: Three exercises—incline dumbbell bench press, lat pulldown (or pullup), and leg press—are arranged in a circuit. Do a set of each, with no rest in between sets, then rest for 2 minutes.

After you've done three circuits, rest for 2 minutes. Then do as many pushups as you can, and rest for 2 minutes. Next, do as many pullups as you can, or do a set of 6 to 8 lat pulldowns, followed by a drop set of as many reps as you can with 20 percent less weight. Rest for 2 minutes, then do leg presses the same way: a set of 6 to 8, followed by as many reps as possible with 20 percent less weight.

INTEGRITY ROUTINE

The exercises are arranged as trisets, which, as you learned in Phase 2, means you do a set of each of them without resting in between. After your first triset, rest for 2 minutes, then do another triset, rest, and do a third triset. You're only going through this workout one time, so you have to put out near-maximal effort in each set to get the desired effect. The workout designates 8 to 12 reps per set, so make sure you choose a weight that you probably can't lift 13 times.

Time

As in the first phase, you should finish all your workouts in well under an hour.

Warmup

CORE ROUTINE

Fat-loss workout: It's a good idea to start out with 5 minutes of general activity—walking, calisthenics, et cetera—before tackling the circuits. Then use the first two circuits as specific warmups. Use light weight the first time through, then slightly heavier weight the second time through, then serious weight the final two times.

Strength workout: Use your first two circuits as warmups. For your first circuit, use one-third of your work-set weight. For the second

circuit, use two-thirds. Then do the other three circuits with your work-set weight.

Muscle workout: Do two warmup circuits, as described for the strength program. Use about 50 percent of your work-set weight in the first warmup set, and about 75 percent in the second.

INTEGRITY ROUTINE

Before starting your workout, try one warmup set of each of the six nonabdominal exercises: leg press, lying leg curl, dumbbell shoulder press, lat pulldown, rope triceps pushdown, and biceps curl. Do six reps of each with two-thirds to three-fourths of your work-set weight.

Speed

In the fat-loss and muscle programs, maintain a deliberate pace—probably 1 second to lift the weights, 2 to 3 seconds to lower them. For strength, lift the weights as fast as you can with good form, and lower them with control.

In the integrity routine, lift at the same deliberate pace you'd use for the fat-loss or muscle routine.

Rest

This is particular to each individual workout, as described earlier, in the initial description of each routine.

Cardiovascular Routine

I'll give detailed instructions after the weight routines, on page 141.

CORE WORKOUT: MONDAYS AND FRIDAYS MAXIMUM FAT LOSS

Exercises	Reps	Week 1	Week 1	Week 2	Week 2	Week 3	Week 3
		Weight/Reps	Weight/Reps	Weight/Reps	Weight/Reps	Weight/Reps	Weight/Reps
CIRCUIT 1 (warmup sets with light weight)							
Squat-and-press	10–12						
Cardio interval (2 min)							
Bent-over row	10–12						
Dumbbell bench press	10–12						
Cardio interval (3 min)							
CIRCUIT 2 (warmup sets with medium weight)							
Squat-and-press	10–12						
Cardio interval (2 min)							
Bent-over row	10–12						
Dumbbell bench press	10–12						
Cardio interval (3 min)							
CIRCUIT 3 (work sets)							
Squat-and-press	10–12						
Cardio interval (2 min)							
Bent-over row	10–12						
Dumbbell bench press	10–12						
Cardio interval (3 min)							
CIRCUIT 4 (work sets)							
Squat-and-press	10–12						
Cardio interval (2 min)							
Bent-over row	10–12						
Dumbbell bench press	10–12						
Cardio interval (3 min)							

CORE WORKOUT: MONDAYS AND FRIDAYS
MAXIMUM STRENGTH

Exercises	Reps	Week 1	Week 1	Week 2	Week 2	Week 3	Week 3
		Weight/Reps	Weight/Reps	Weight/Reps	Weight/Reps	Weight/Reps	Weight/Reps
CIRCUIT 1 (warmup sets with ⅓ of work-set weight)							
Deadlift	4–6						
Rest (2 min)							
Dumbbell bench press	3–5						
Squat	4–6						
Rest (3 min)							
CIRCUIT 2 (warmup sets with ⅔ of work-set weight)							
Deadlift	4–6						
Rest (2 min)							
Dumbbell bench press	3–5						
Squat	4–6						
Rest (3 min)							
CIRCUIT 3 (work sets)							
Deadlift	4–6						
Rest (2 min)							
Dumbbell bench press	3–5						
Squat	4–6						
Rest (3 min)							
CIRCUIT 4 (work sets)							
Deadlift	4–6						
Rest (2 min)							
Dumbbell bench press	3–5						
Squat	4–6						
Rest (3 min)							
CIRCUIT 5 (work sets)							
Deadlift	4–6						
Rest (2 min)							
Dumbbell bench press	3–5						
Squat	4–6						
Rest (3 min)							

CORE WORKOUT: MONDAYS AND FRIDAYS
MAXIMUM MUSCLE

Exercises	Reps	Week 1	Week 1	Week 2	Week 2	Week 3	Week 3
		Weight/Reps	Weight/Reps	Weight/Reps	Weight/Reps	Weight/Reps	Weight/Reps
CIRCUIT 1 (warmup sets with 1/2 of work-set weight)							
Incline dumbbell bench press	4–6						
Lat pulldown (or pullup)	3–5						
Leg press	4–6						
Rest (2 min)							
CIRCUIT 2 (warmup sets with 3/4 of work-set weight)							
Incline dumbbell bench press	4–6						
Lat pulldown (or pullup)	3–5						
Leg press	4–6						
Rest (2 min)							
CIRCUIT 3 (work sets)							
Incline dumbbell bench press	4–6						
Lat pulldown (or pullup)	3–5						
Leg press	4–6						
Rest (2 min)							
Pushup	Burnout						
Rest (2 min)							
Lat pulldown (or pullup)							
Set 1	6–8 (or burnout)						
Set 2 (drop)*	Burnout						
Rest (2 min)							
Leg press							
Set 1	6–8						
Set 2 (drop)	Burnout						

* Lat pulldown only, not pullup

INTEGRITY WORKOUT: WEDNESDAYS

Exercise	Reps	Week 1	Week 2	Week 3
		Weight/Reps	Weight/Reps	Weight/Reps
TRISET 1				
Leg press	8–12			
Lying leg curl	8–12			
Swiss-ball reverse crunch	8–12			
Rest (2 min)				
TRISET 2				
Dumbbell shoulder press	8–12			
Lat pulldown	8–12			
Swiss-ball reverse crunch	8–12			
Rest (2 min)				
TRISET 3				
Rope triceps pushdown	8–12			
Biceps curl	8–12			
Swiss-ball reverse crunch	8–12			

Cardiovascular-Training Workout

BEGINNER ROUTINE
If you haven't done any cardiovascular exercise in the past 6 months, try the beginner routine in Phase 1 (see page 88).

ADVANCED ROUTINE
If you've done the advanced cardiovascular-training workouts in Phases 1, 2, and 3, try this high-intensity interval routine.

Using any type of aerobic exercise, perform each sprint described at right at the prescribed percentage of your highest possible effort (see "Rating Your Cardio Effort" on page 88 to determine each percentage).

Warm up for 5 minutes.

→ Sprint for 2 minutes at 80 percent of your highest possible effort.

→ Throttle down to 45 percent of your maximum effort for 2 minutes.

→ Do these 80 percent–45 percent intervals a total of three times.

→ Cool down for 3 minutes at about 50 percent of full effort.

The Exercises

SQUAT-AND-PRESS

1 Grab a pair of dumbbells and stand holding them just outside your shoulders, with your arms bent and your palms facing each other. Set your feet shoulder-width apart; keep your back straight, your knees slightly bent, and your eyes focused straight ahead.

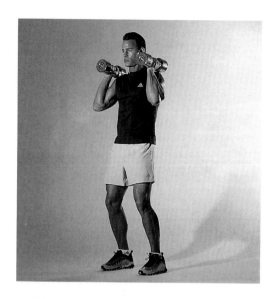

2 Keeping your back in its natural alignment and your lower legs nearly perpendicular to the floor, slowly lower your body as if you were sitting back into a chair. When your thighs are parallel to the floor, pause.

3 Press your feet off the floor to push yourself back up to the starting position while you press the weights over your head. Lower the weights and repeat.

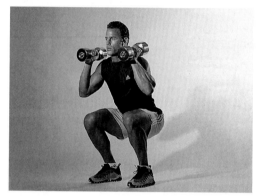

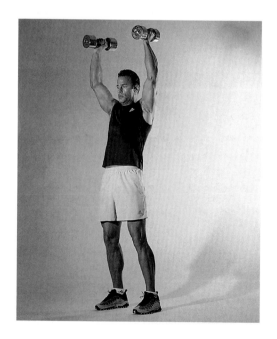

BENT-OVER ROW

1 Grab a barbell with an overhand grip that's just beyond shoulder-width, and hold it at arm's length. Stand with your feet shoulder-width apart and your knees slightly bent. Bend at the hips, lowering your torso about 45 degrees, and let the bar hang straight down from your shoulders.

2 Pull the bar up to your torso. Pause, then slowly lower it.

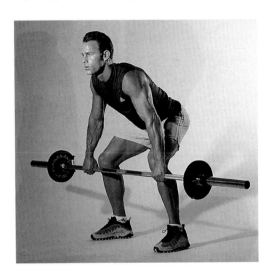
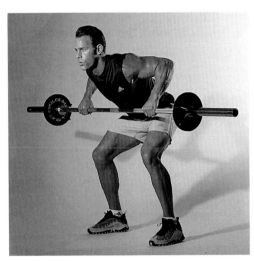

DUMBBELL BENCH PRESS

1 Grab a pair of dumbbells and lie faceup on a flat bench. Hold the dumbbells just outside your shoulders, with your arms bent and your palms facing your feet.

2 Push the weights up and slightly inward so that when your arms are extended, the dumbbells are above your collarbones. Lower the weights back to your chest, and pause before repeating.

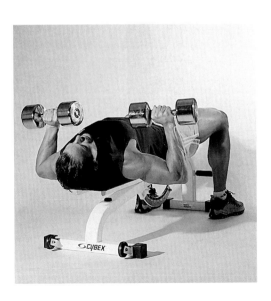
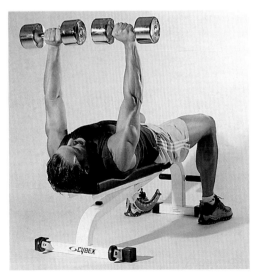

DEADLIFT

1 Roll a barbell against your shins. Grab the bar with an overhand grip, your hands just beyond shoulder-width. Squat down, focus your eyes straight ahead, and pull your shoulders back.

2 Stand with the bar, thrusting your hips forward and keeping your shoulders pulled back. Pause, then slowly lower the bar to the floor, keeping it as close to your body as possible. When you bring the bar down past your knees, squat down, rather than bend forward at the waist.

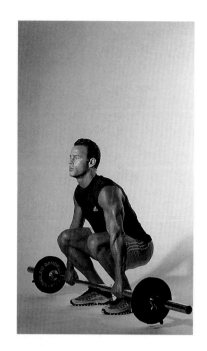
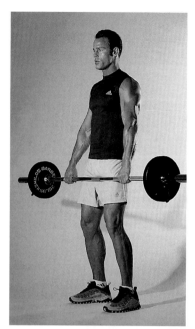

SQUAT

1 Set a barbell on a squat rack and step under it so the bar rests across your upper back. Pull your shoulders back as you grab the bar with an overhand grip. The bar should sit comfortably on your upper trapezius muscles. Lift the bar off the rack and step back. Set your feet shoulder-width apart; keep your back straight, your knees slightly bent, and your eyes focused straight ahead.

2 Slowly lower your body as if you were sitting back into a chair, keeping your back in its natural alignment and your lower legs nearly perpendicular to the floor. When your thighs are parallel to the floor, pause before returning to the starting position.

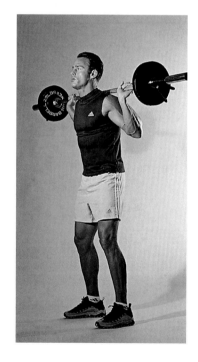
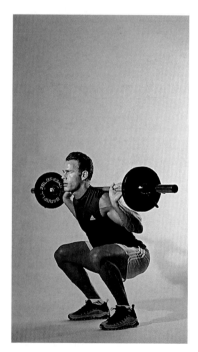

INCLINE DUMBBELL BENCH PRESS

1 Adjust a bench to a 10- to 30-degree incline. Grab a pair of dumbbells and sit on the bench. Hold the dumbbells just outside your shoulders, with your arms bent and your palms facing forward.

2 Push the weights up and slightly inward so that when your arms are extended, the dumbbells are above your collarbones. Lower the weights back to your chest, and pause before repeating.

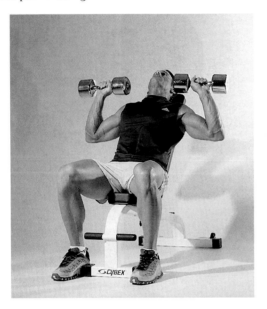

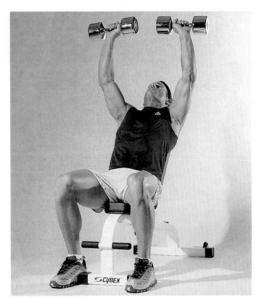

LAT PULLDOWN

1 Sit at a lat-pulldown station and grab the bar with a "false" overhand grip that's just beyond shoulder-width. A false grip means you place your thumb on top of the bar, alongside your index finger, rather than wrap it around the bar.

2 Pull the bar down to your chest. Pause, then slowly return to the starting position.

If you don't have access to this machine: Do a pullover with dumbbells. Lie faceup on a bench and hold the weights over your chest with your arms extended, your elbows slightly bent, and your palms facing your toes. The weights should be perpendicular to the floor. Keeping your back flat against the bench to elongate your lats, slowly lower the weights behind your head until your upper arms are parallel to the floor. Keep a slight bend in your elbows throughout. Then pull back to the starting position.

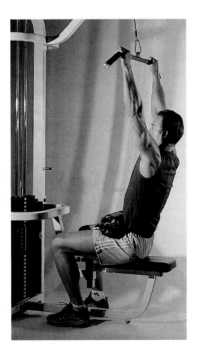

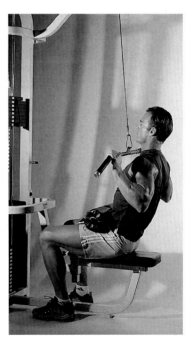

PULLUP

1 Grab a pullup bar with an overhand grip, your hands just outside shoulder-width. Hang at arm's length with your knees bent and your feet crossed behind you.

2 Pull yourself up until your chin passes the bar. Pause, then slowly lower yourself.

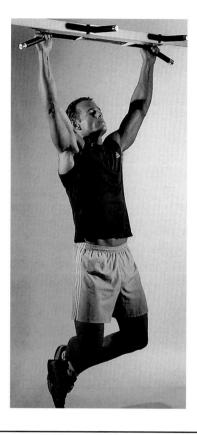
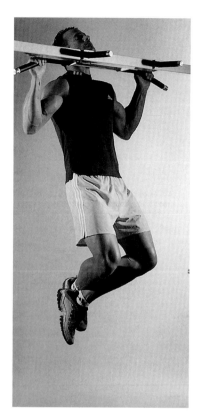

LEG PRESS

1 Position yourself in the leg-press machine so that your back is against the pad and your feet are about hip-width apart on the platform.

2 Unlock the platform, and slowly lower the weights until your knees are bent 90 degrees. Pause, then push back up to the starting position.

If you don't have access to this machine: Do squats, described on page 144, instead.

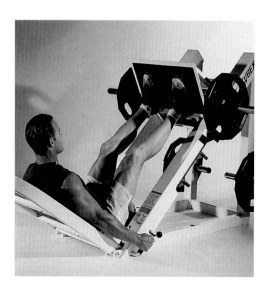
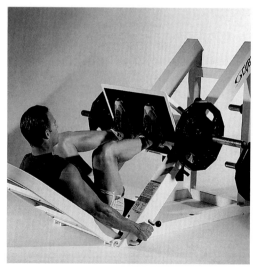

PUSHUP

1 Position yourself facedown on the floor, with your weight supported on your hands and toes. Your hands should be shoulder-width apart, fingers pointed forward. Your feet should be hip-width apart. Keep your arms, back, and legs straight.

2 Bend at the elbows to slowly lower yourself to the floor. Stop when your chest is an inch from the floor, pause, then push yourself back up to the starting position.

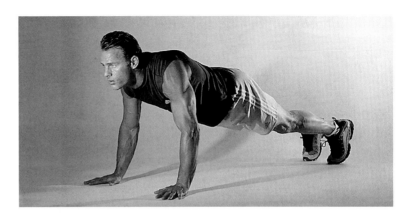

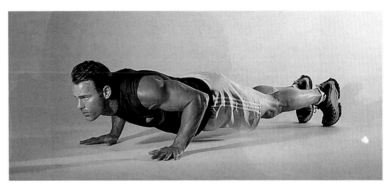

LYING LEG CURL

1 Lie on the leg-curl machine with the pads against your lower legs, above your heels and below your calf muscles.

2 Without raising your hips off the bench, bend your legs at the knees and pull the weight toward your butt as far as you can. Pause, then slowly return to the starting position.

If you don't have access to this machine: Do the exercise lying on a bench, holding a dumbbell between your feet.

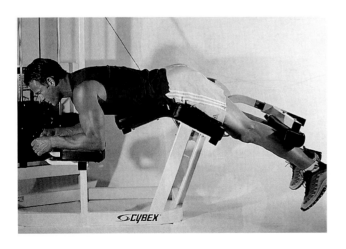

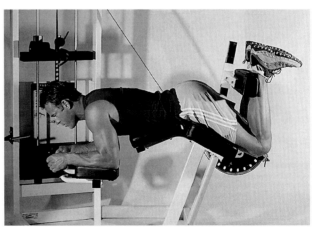

SWISS-BALL REVERSE CRUNCH

1 Lie faceup on a slant board, with your hips lower than your head. Grab the bar behind your head for support. Bend your hips and knees at 90-degree angles and hold a small Swiss ball between your hamstrings and your calves. Start with your butt flat against the board.

2 Pull your hips up and in toward your rib cage, as if emptying a bucket of water that was resting on your pelvis. Curl them as high as you can without lifting your shoulders off the board, and keep your hips and knees at 90-degree angles. Pause, then slowly return to the starting position. If this exercise is too difficult, perform it on the floor or without the Swiss ball.

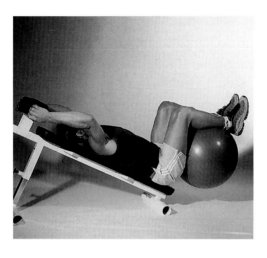
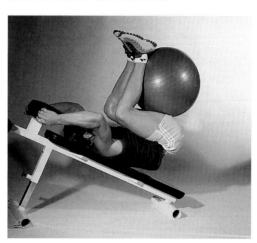

DUMBBELL SHOULDER PRESS

1 Grab a pair of dumbbells and sit holding them just outside your shoulders, with your arms bent and your palms facing each other.

2 Push the weights straight overhead. Pause, then slowly lower them.

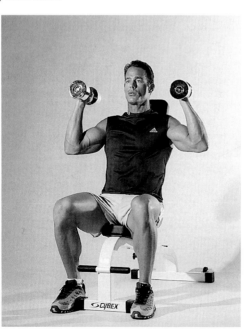
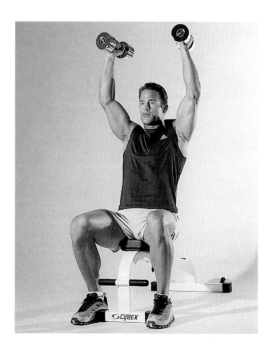

ROPE TRICEPS PUSHDOWN

1 Attach a rope handle to the high pulley of a cable station and grab it so your palms face each other. Start with your elbows bent 90 degrees and your upper arms against your sides.

2 Straighten your arms, allowing your hands to pull the rope ends outward at the bottom. Pause, then slowly return to the starting position.

If you don't have access to this machine: Do a seated dumbbell triceps extension. Grab a pair of dumbbells and sit on a bench or chair. Hold the dumbbells overhead with straight arms. Bend at the elbows to slowly lower the weights behind and to the sides of your head. Hold your upper arms in the same position. Pause, then push up to the starting position.

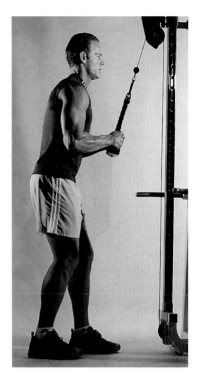
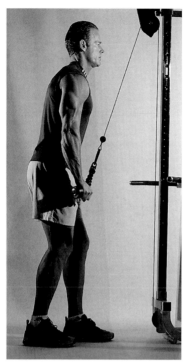

BICEPS CURL

1 Grab an EZ-curl bar with an underhand, shoulder-width grip. Stand with your feet staggered so your left foot is in front of you; keep your knees slightly bent and your back straight. Hold the bar at arm's length, in front of your thighs. Keep your upper arms tucked against your sides.

2 Curl the bar as high as you can without letting your upper arms move forward. Pause, then slowly return to the starting position.

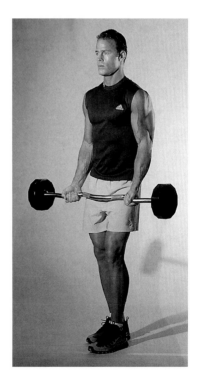
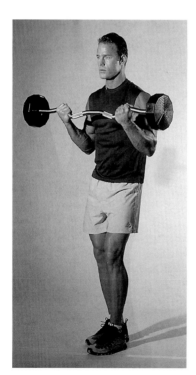

PART THREE

THE
LEANING
CURVE

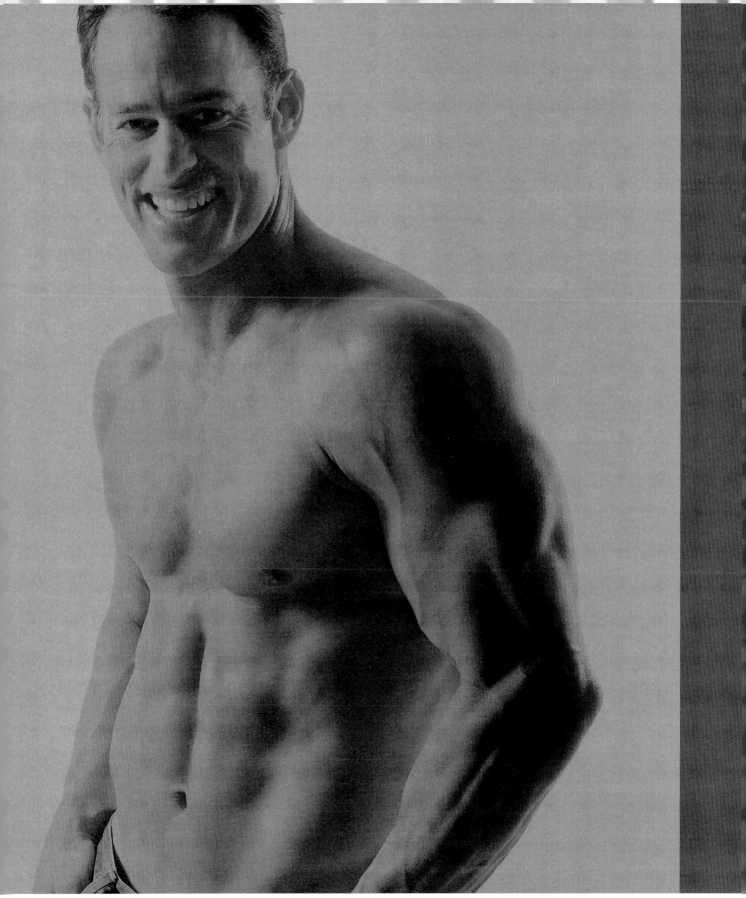

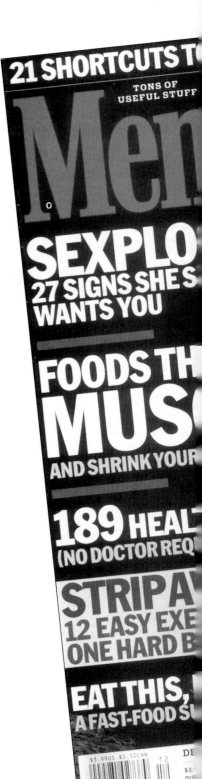

21 SHORTCUTS T

TONS OF
USEFUL STUFF

Men

SEXPLO
27 SIGNS SHE S
WANTS YOU

FOODS TH
MUSC
AND SHRINK YOUR

189 HEAL
(NO DOCTOR REQ

STRIP A
12 EASY EXE
ONE HARD B

EAT THIS,
A FAST-FOOD S

DE

$3.99US $5.50CAN   12

$3.
DIS

09281 02737 9

II
A

LEAN, BUT NEVER HUNGRY

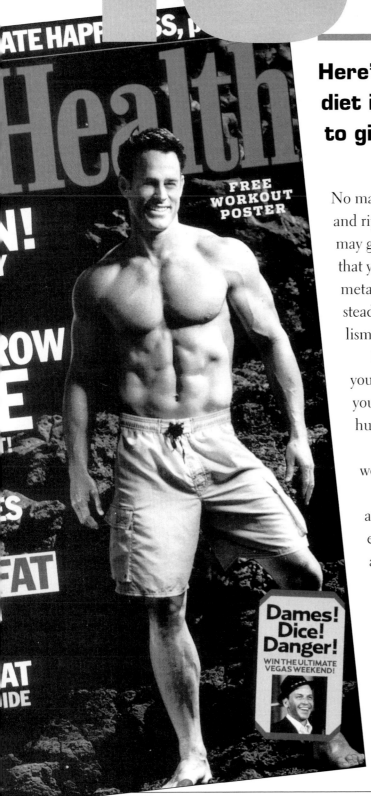

Here's the most important diet information I'm going to give you: You must eat.

No matter how jacked up you are about getting lean and ripped, you won't help yourself by starving. You may get leaner for a few hours, maybe a day, but after that your body compensates by slowing down your metabolism. Conversely, when you give your body a steady supply of clean-burning fuel, your metabolism stays up and running smoothly.

In order to lose enough fat to achieve the look you want, you must find a meal plan that allows you to eat consistently and never leaves you feeling hungry or deprived.

The second-most-important lesson is this: You won't achieve your goals with a crash diet.

I know that some guys reading this book have a lot of weight to lose. And I know that if you're excited about starting the program, you're probably thinking, "Why not lose weight fast?"

Again, there's the metabolic issue. Rapid weight loss almost always includes a reduction in muscle as well as in fat. When you lose muscle, your metabolism slows. If you starve yourself on a crash diet, you slow it down even more.

Lost muscle produces another nasty side effect: The less muscle you have, and the slower your metabolism, the easier it is to re-gain weight. And guess what that weight is going to be? Fat. So then you have more fat to lose, in addition to the handicap of a slower metabolism.

The flip side of all this is the program I recommend: food, and lots of it. Yup, you heard it. Eat! If you want to lose weight, that is . . . If you've ever believed that eating lots of food and losing fat are actions at odds with each other, forget it. They're not just compatible; they're bedfellows.

Food is more than raw material for your muscles, more than energy for your workouts. It's essential to maintaining your metabolism, your daily physical and mental functions, and the integrity of your cellular structures.

Of course, there's food, and then there's food eaten according to a larger plan. Rest assured, though, that this will probably be the least complicated diet plan you're ever going to get. I'm not a big believer in complex meal charts and chemical breakdowns. I respect the science, but simple guidelines and common sense will get the job done if you're consistent about implementing them.

In this chapter and the next, I'm going to give you my guidelines for an eating program you can follow day in and day out. There's no food involved that you can't buy at your local grocery store. You can take this diet with you to restaurants. And you can follow it for life.

All you need to bring to the table is a determination to consistently eat right.

"When it comes to diet, I tend to have the most success when I use my eyeballs and common sense."

It's Not Just What You Eat That Matters—It's When

You should eat about every 3 waking hours. That works out to five small-to-medium-size meals a day, or three meals and two snacks. I don't care what you call them, just so long as you eat something every 3 hours. Ideally, eat something that contains at least two of the three macronutrients: protein, fat, and carbohydrates. So one of the snacks could be a smoothie made with protein powder. That gives you carbohydrate and, obviously, protein. Or you could have peanut butter and an apple—that gives you protein, carbohydrate, and fat.

If you've read a lot of diet and exercise books, you've probably seen a plan like this in every one. I don't pretend mine is unique, but I do guarantee that it works. Why? First, it prevents you from overeating. When you don't eat all day—like from noon to 7:00 P.M.—you get home and feel like you could eat a horse. So you eat a lot, and you eat it fast. By the time your body registers that you've eaten anything (this usually takes about 20 minutes), you've eaten more than you wanted to.

If you eat regularly throughout the day, you don't get that sensation of ravenous, out-of-control hunger. Often, you eat before you're hungry at all. That makes it easy to exert control over your diet. You know when you're going to eat, and you have plenty of time to decide what you're going to eat. You never put yourself in a position in which you have to eat whatever's in front of you. And there you have the two keys to healthy eating: You decide what you're going to eat, and you have enough discipline to know what you're not going to eat.

A lot of people balk at the idea of eating five times a day instead of three, thinking that five meals must add up to more calories than the three meals they're already eating. In fact, though, the opposite is true. When you eat five times a day, and often eat before you feel any hunger at all, you can eat less at every meal—sometimes substantially less. Five 500-calorie meals can feel like more food than three 1,000-calorie meals.

The biggest challenge may be juggling your schedule to accommodate the extra meals. Many businesses, most families, and all prisons are set up around the three-meal model. In those situations, meal-replacement bars come in handy. Go for the ones designed for bodybuilders, which have plenty of protein and comparatively few carbohydrates. Avoid the ones for endurance athletes, which are mostly carbohydrates. And whatever you do, stay away from the cereal bars. Those are virtually all carbohydrates, and they're so quickly digested that the net effect is probably to stimulate your appetite, rather than sate it.

The Night Is a Different World

You'll be amazed at the progress you'll make if you just change your evening eating habits. You still have to eat at night—you don't ever want to go to bed hungry—but two smart adjustments can cut your nighttime calories dramatically.

First, stop thinking of dinner as your biggest meal of the day. In my experience, lean people tend to front-load their calories, eating more of them earlier in the day and tapering off at night. Dinner can still be a time for the family to be together. Or it can still be the centerpiece of your dating strategy, if that's your style. But it doesn't have to be a big meal.

Second, avoid starchy carbohydrates in the evening. I try not to eat any "dry carbs"—rice, pasta, potatoes, or any kind of bread—after 4:00 P.M. That may be too strict a guideline for you, and if there's anything I've learned in my many years of giving advice to anyone who asks, it's that people can't make sweeping, radical changes to their lives just because I tell them to. Each guy has to experiment and see what works best in his life.

"A healthy, lean, active body needs all three macronutrients: protein, carbohydrates, and fat."

But I will say this: The better you can control your dry-carb intake throughout the day, and the fewer dry carbs you eat in the evening, the faster you will see results from this program.

So now that you know what to avoid for dinner, here's what I suggest instead: lean meat (without the potato) or fish (without the rice), along with green vegetables or a salad. You need some fat in this meal, which can come in the form of olive oil on the vegetables, nuts and dressing on the salad, or in a pesto sauce on the meat or fish.

This is probably a lot like what you're eating now. In fact, I'm asking you to make only three changes.

1. Eat early and often throughout the day, including a mid-afternoon meal or snack, so you won't be ravenous at dinnertime.

2. Avoid dry carbs.

3. Drink plenty of water.

That's it. You have half of the cover model diet mastered already. Try this for one or two nights, and I guarantee your belly will be flatter in the morning. Do it consistently, and you'll be a lean machine in a matter of months.

My way: Give me a steady fuel line and a cup of joe. I'm often asked about what to eat before exercise. Nobody wants to settle for plain-jane unleaded if there's a premium pre-workout fuel they can ingest instead. A lot of guys have heard about the carbo-loading that marathoners and other endurance athletes indulge in before a competition. And if they've been paying attention, they know about the new research showing that pre-workout protein can enhance post-workout muscle building.

I don't like a lot of carbs or a lot of protein before a workout. The only thing I ever consume just before a workout is coffee. Coffee is the one vice left over from my party days. But I don't consider it a vice in this context. Java is a superb energizer with a lot of other health benefits. A triple cappuccino does more for my workout than any plate of pasta or chicken breast I've ever had.

If you eat every 3 hours, as I urge you to do, you won't be exercising on an empty carb tank. You'll also get plenty of protein throughout the day to build muscle mass. Marathoners are trying to survive—they need to load up on carbohydrates. You don't. Body-builders who eat protein before their workouts are trying to bulk up. You aren't.

If you absolutely can't work out without

eating a little something on the way to the gym, I guess a banana or an apple is okay. But I think you'll be better off if you time your meals so your workout falls between two of them. So eat an hour or two before a workout, and then immediately or soon afterward.

That keeps you on both programs—exercise and diet—without disrupting either. And I think you'll find, as I do, that it's better to fuel workout from the energy pipeline you've already established, rather than create a new one.

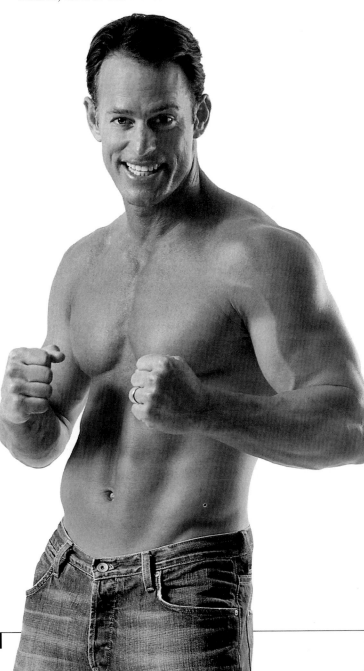

Of course, there's nothing like a cup of coffee to put a little more heat on that fuel.

Protein: The Raw Material of a Cover Model Body

A healthy, lean, active body needs all three macronutrients: protein, carbohydrates, and fat. Each plays multiple roles, and all those roles are important. But I'm going to talk about protein first because I think it's the hardest to get right. We live in a world of cheap carbohydrates and hidden fats. You get those things in foods, whether you want them or not. But you need to seek out high-quality protein. Building your diet around it requires deliberate effort.

"Your muscles are mostly water, but the parts that aren't water are built with protein."

The first role of protein is building your muscles. I'm sure you already know that, but it's worth emphasizing. Your muscles are mostly water, but the parts that aren't water are built with protein. Your workouts break down protein in your muscles but also trigger the process that ultimately leads to bigger, stronger muscles, as your body lays down new protein to replace the old.

How much protein do you need? The science is pretty clear. A guy who's doing a lot of strength training needs an estimated 1.6 to 1.8 grams of protein per kilogram of body weight, each day. That's about 0.7 to 0.8 gram per pound. So if you weigh 200 pounds, you want to eat 140 to 160 grams a day.

A lot of people say a lot of disparaging things about protein. Seems like every day, some official organization levels a new attack on a "high-protein diet," mainly to keep Dr. Atkins from selling books. These people say you can get by on very little protein—50 grams a day, or something like that.

I won't debate them on the science. If they're talking about people who don't do any exercise at all, I'll take their word for it. But "getting by" isn't good enough for me or anyone I know. If you're reading this book, you should be a regular exerciser or prepared to become one. So the minimum amounts of protein required for survival aren't nearly good enough for you.

There's another side to this argument: recommending more protein. Some say a gram a pound is better. For me, that would be about 200 grams a day (when you see me on a cover, I usually weigh about 190 pounds, but my average weight between shoots is about 200). I find I gain too much muscle with that intake. I know, I know, it's a problem most guys would love to have. And believe me, I'm not complaining about it. I'm just saying that I look and feel best with a little less.

A higher-protein diet poses a health risk only if you have a preexisting kidney illness. If you don't have one of those, there's no evidence that a higher protein intake is harmful. And there is some evidence that higher protein—about 25 percent of total calories—is healthier than lower protein. People lose more weight on higher protein, and have less heart disease.

I recommend dividing your protein almost evenly among your five meals. So if you're shooting for 150 grams a day (just to pick a nice round number), you'll be looking at 30 grams five times a day. How much is 30 grams?

→ 5 eggs
→ 3 ounces of lean meat (a serving about the size of a deck of cards)
→ 4 to 6 ounces of fish
→ 1½ scoops of whey protein powder

Here are a few foods you can combine to get 30 grams.

→ 1 cup of low-fat cottage cheese (9 grams)
→ 1 cup of 2% milk (8 grams)
→ 2 tablespoons of peanut butter, or a serving about the size of a golf ball (7 grams)
→ 2 slices of whole wheat bread (6 grams)

Now, I'm going to make a terrible confession: I don't spend my days weighing and measuring food. You might want to, but you may not. I believe that you do have to be very precise about your exercise program—keeping track of every set and rep—if you're going to make progress. But when it comes to diet, I tend to have the most success when I use my eyeballs and common sense.

You may be different. I know studies have shown that keeping food logs helps dieters. One study even showed that people who kept food diaries over the holidays actually lost weight, whereas most people gain a little weight between Thanksgiving and New Year's. So if you think a log will help you keep track of things, go for it.

At the same time, I think there's a lot to be said for simple consistency in your meals. And one great way to establish consistency is to build each meal around a baseline amount of protein. *My way: Eat lots of chicken, turkey,*

and fish, since animal proteins deliver the most protein per ounce and have been shown to be the best muscle builders. (If you're a vegetarian, you have to work a little harder to get your protein, but you can do it. I like to include soy and all kinds of beans in my diet. I'm also big on nuts, if they're fresh and unsalted.)

I also go for a whey-protein shake just about every day. I have a shake for breakfast when I'm on the run, or as my post-workout, mid-morning meal.

Carbohydrates: Smart Fuel for Your Workouts

I have to confess that I have no idea what happens to your body when you don't eat carbohydrates. I've read that carbs are not essential nutrients—your body can survive without them, though it needs protein and fat. But I've never been tempted to explore the carb-free life. Mainly because I don't need to. The diet I eat now—which includes plenty of carbs—keeps me lean and healthy, so I'm going to stick with it.

Carbohydrates are your body's preferred source of fuel. They're stored in your muscles, where they're ready to help you whenever you want to move. During prolonged exercise, they help you burn fat. Exercise scientists like to say that fat burns in a carbohydrate flame. Though fat is your body's best source of energy, carbohydrates make it possible to use that fat.

The thing about carbohydrates is that different types have very different effects on your body. I've already told you to stay away from dry carbs most of the time, especially at night. Those foods, in my view, are easy to overeat and, unless you're a competitive athlete, give you far more fuel than you need.

On the other hand, vegetables—dark, fiber-rich carbs—have the opposite effect. They don't contain many calories, and they aren't as easy to eat or as tasty as bread and pasta. So eating too much asparagus, broccoli, lettuce, brussels sprouts, spinach, and green beans will never be a problem. Eating enough of them is the bigger issue, as any parent will tell you. If your mom has said "Eat your vegetables" once, she's probably said it hundreds of times.

The fiber in vegetables has amazing health benefits—it's been linked to weight control, heart health, and disease prevention. Fiber-rich foods help you feel satisfied during a meal, as does protein, so you stop eating sooner. That helps explain why fiber and protein are so crucial to weight control. A rule to live by: If you can control your weight, you control your health.

Way on the other end of the nutritional spectrum are the simple sugars and sweeteners, such as sucrose (table sugar) and high-fructose corn syrup. These products are, for lack of a better term, pure evil. Some intriguing new research shows that your body has a hard time detecting fructose sweeteners in your stomach. So the signals that normally tell you that you've eaten fail to kick in. If you don't believe me, try this experiment: Next time you're hungry, drink a 12-ounce Coke or Mountain Dew. Even better, drink two. I bet you'll still find yourself hungry, despite the fact that you'll have just taken in about 300 calories. You'll have given your body fuel, but your hunger-sating mechanisms won't realize it.

My way: Stay away from sugar and sugar alcohol. The word *sugar* has different meanings for different people. I consider any quickly digesting carbohydrate to be a sugar, since that's how my body treats it after I eat. So when I eat a potato or a slice of white bread, in my mind I may as well be eating a packet of pure, granulated sucrose.

In this area, I have the same temptations as anyone else. I mean, I have a child, and where there are children, there is cake. My strategy is to eat sweets on an empty stomach, with plenty of water. That way, I don't pile empty calories on top of the calories from other food.

You may hear some bodybuilder types talk about avoiding fruit because of the simple sugars. But with fruit, the good far outweighs the bad. The sugars in fruit don't act as fast as the sugar in that cake, since the fiber they contain slows them down. The fiber also has the same health benefits that the fiber in vegetables does. Fruit's vitamins and minerals have a lengthy list of proven benefits as well. So I love eating fruit. To me, it's one of the joys of being alive. Fruit is God's edible version of flowers. I think it's unnatural to *not* eat it.

I throw fruit into all my shakes and smoothies, and have yet to detect any damage to my waistline. I do, however, draw the line at fruit juices. When you take the fiber out of fruit, you still get the vitamins and antioxidants, but you create a product that's much more like table sugar. It hits your bloodstream fast, and the faster a food goes through your system, the sooner you get hungry again.

"Carbohydrates are your body's preferred source of fuel."

So eat fruit when you're hungry, and drink water when you're thirsty. Or better yet, eat fruit before you're hungry, and drink water before you're thirsty.

As for beer and wine, I put them in the same category as sweets. Sugar alcohol isn't technically a nutrient. Your body tries so hard to get rid of it that it processes it preferentially, before any food you eat simultaneously. And your body burns so many calories trying to get rid of it that if you have alcohol without food, the net effect is that you burn more calories metabolically than you take in from the alcohol. So alcohol would be the perfect weight-loss beverage if it didn't waste your muscles, cause your body to store extra fat in your belly, rot your liver, and give you the green light to tell your boss what you really think of his management techniques.

Again, I'm no saint, and I'm not telling you to be one. If you like an occasional beer, have an occasional beer. But if the beer is more than occasional, you can forget about having a lean physique.

When you do have wine or beer with a meal, consider it your carbohydrate. Have two beers and a steak, and you can survive with your physique intact. A six-pack with pizza will set you back.

And, although I sound like a broken record, remember to drink plenty of water before, during, and after.

Fat: A Key Part of the Mix

Don't fall for the myth that dietary fat is nothing but evil. Your body needs it. Your brain is about 70 percent fat; your manliest hormone, testosterone, is made from fat; and fat is vital to your body's cellular structures.

A low-fat diet is a bad idea for most people. Not only that, it's nearly impossible to stick with. You put your psyche through hell, for very little benefit. Your body is smart. It won't let go of the fat it has if it's convinced that no more is coming. You may lose some body fat early in a low-fat diet program, but in the long run your body finds a way to compensate, creating fat out of the carbohydrates you eat. That's why I believe in giving your body the fat it needs.

To my mind, some of the worst dietary choices you can make are low-fat or fat-free versions of desserts that normally have some fat in them. These foods usually have just as many calories, with sugar replacing the fat to give the food substance.

My way: Go for the friendly fats.
There's fat, and then there's fat. My diet includes a lot of monounsaturated fats, the type found in nuts, olive oil, peanut butter, and avocados. I also seek out foods with omega-3 polyunsaturated fats, found in fish and fish oil.

I try to minimize saturated fats, the ones found in meat and dairy foods. Saturated fats raise cholesterol levels—not what a guy like me, who's fighting a bad-heart gene, needs. Fortunately, most meats are leaner now than they were decades ago. And some cuts—such as those with *strip* or *loin* in their names—are relatively lean to begin with. When I have dairy foods such as milk and yogurt, I go for the low-fat versions.

"I believe in giving your body the fat it needs."

One type of fat I avoid at all costs is trans fat, found in baked goods, fried foods, and margarine.

I confess that none of this is simple or instinctual. You have to read labels, and even then the labels tell only half the story. There's a move to force companies to list how many grams of trans fats are in different foods. They already have to tell you how much saturated fat is in food. But even when you know all that, you still don't know much about the other fats.

For example, mayonnaise doesn't have much saturated fat, but it has lots of soybean oil, a type of polyunsaturated fat called omega-6. Foods today are full of omega-6's, though a lot of experts now think these fats cause inflammation that can lead to health problems—including major ones such as heart disease and Alzheimer's.

Ice cream is another dangerous food since it combines saturated fat with lots of sugar.

As complicated as all this seems, however, you can rely on your common sense much of the time. I mean, do you really need me to tell you that scarfing down a chicken-fried steak and a pint of Ben & Jerry's isn't going to get you a cover-caliber body?

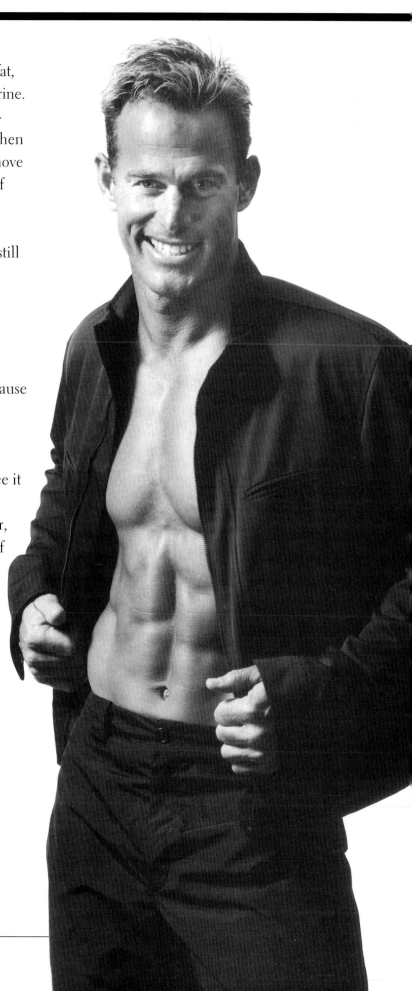

THE COVER MODEL DIET

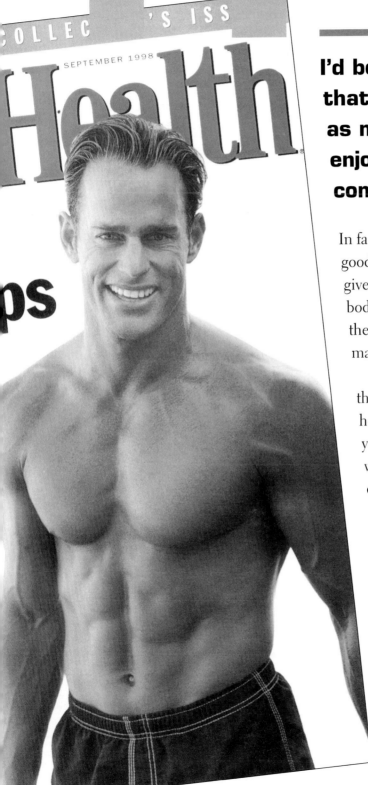

COLLEC   'S ISS

SEPTEMBER 1998

Health

I'd be willing to wager that I enjoy my healthy diet as much as other guys enjoy their so-called comfort food.

In fact, I probably enjoy it more. It not only tastes good to me but also makes me feel great. Plus, it gives me the satisfaction of knowing I'm giving my body the food that will result in terrific workouts and the lean physique that's been my calling card for so many years.

You won't suffer on the Cover Model Diet. To the contrary, you'll rediscover the pleasure of hearty, guilt-free eating. But for that to happen, you have to adjust your attitude. You have to always be aware that what you put inside your body determines how it looks from the outside. Not only that, it determines how you feel.

Food doesn't exist just to please your palate and satisfy your hunger. Its main purpose is to fuel and build your body. But here's a weird thing I've discovered about eating for performance, rather than for pleasure: The pleasure of eating actually increases when you stop eating for pleasure. This is yet another way that clean living becomes a self-perpetuating phenomenon.

The Diet You Like versus the Diet That Likes You

I know that the hardest part of shifting to a diet that will get you into the best possible condition is the thought of "giving up" some foods you've always loved. Most of us were brought up with potatoes on the plate with our steaks, with jelly on our toast, with cake or ice cream as a reward for eating a few vegetables without gagging.

You can rest easy. Never in a million years would I advise you to immediately and permanently swear off any food you like. You wouldn't listen to me if I did. More important, it's not a smart thing to try to do.

First of all, a lot of suspect foods don't need to be completely eliminated—and probably shouldn't be. You know how down I am on dry carbs such as potatoes, bread, and rice? Well, in a few pages you're going to see that I actually recommend those foods for some meals. It's just a question of rethinking when you eat them and how much of them you consume.

Second, it's pure folly to try to go cold turkey on foods you've loved all your life—even the ones that will never do you any good. You have to wean yourself off those things slowly. It's not that hard to spread a little less butter on your toast each time you eat it, or to lighten up on the salt and start phasing in other spices instead. Just as in your workouts, little steps will get you there.

Finally, nothing is for always. I don't just allow you to indulge yourself with ice cream or a steaming plate of pasta on occasion; I insist on it. You have to splurge now and then, because

you're human. The difference is that your new attitude will make those foods special treats, not everyday necessities. You'll be in control.

Free Yourself of a Bad Habit You Didn't Know You Had

Your task is to get into the habit of eating healthy meals. That also means getting *out* of the habit of eating unhealthy ones. It's easier to do both those things when you realize that a lot of the questionable food choices you've been making are nothing but unconscious routines and assumptions.

> "A lot of the questionable food choices you've been making are nothing but unconscious routines and assumptions."

For example, why would you drink soda with your meals? Probably just because you always have. Yet all you're doing is pouring in sugar and chemicals that upset the macronutrient balance of your meals. This should be an easy habit to phase out. Water quenches your thirst better than any soft drink, and it's one of the best things you can possibly put into your body.

Whole milk was great to grow on when you were a kid, but now you don't need all that saturated fat. Low-fat milk may not taste as good to you at first. But if you make the effort to switch over, pretty soon it's the whole milk that's going to taste bad. Again, it's a question of habit.

Commercial cold cereals that are loaded with sugar and preservatives, with all the natural nutrients and fiber processed out of them, are probably another childhood holdover. You can get used to whole grain cereals with lots of fiber and very little sugar or sodium—even though those are exactly the ones you hated as a kid.

Start questioning your assumptions about which foods you like. You'll feel liberated and more in tune with my eating guidelines. Where is it written, for example, that you have to load up your tuna with mayonnaise to enjoy it? Tuna is a great food for building lean muscle mass and losing fat, and it tastes great by itself. You won't miss the mayo.

I also recommend staying away from ketchup, mustard, soy sauce, tartar sauce, sweet-and-sour sauce, barbecue sauce, and steak sauce. Any spice or herb in your cabinet can be combined with a touch of olive oil for great flavoring. You can sauté tomatoes, onion, and garlic to season your meat. Like everything else in your quest for a great body and optimal health, it's just a matter of replacing bad habits with good ones.

Out with the Old, in with the New

Once you start questioning your age-old assumptions about eating, all kinds of good things can happen. As I mentioned in the previous chapter, a common habit I strongly urge you to break is making your evening meal the biggest of the day. As a model and athlete, I've traveled abroad a lot, and I can tell you that many cultures don't eat that way. You shouldn't either. If you want to lose fat and build muscle, your dinner should be no bigger than your lunch.

Another aforementioned habit you've probably had all your life is eating three meals a day and snacking at random between them. It's much healthier and energy boosting to eat five meals a day, actually planning your snacks as small mid-morning and mid-afternoon meals.

You may also be in the habit of having dessert right after your meal. That's another custom to change for the better. If you must have a sweet dessert, wait at least 40 minutes after a meal. Give your digestive system a chance to process a nicely balanced meal before throwing everything out of whack with a ton of sugar.

Finally, rethink what a meal actually is. You can drink it as well as eat it. I love smoothies, and I fix 'em up so they make a perfect meal, with the right amounts of calories, protein, carbohydrates, and fat. Sometimes I have two or three a day. When you're shooting for a cover-caliber body, smoothies become part of your life.

My way: Don't go to dietary extremes. I'm a dedicated healthy eater, but I'm not half as extreme with my diet as I am with my workouts. My advice to you is to be consistent but not fanatical. Don't *never* have cake, or pasta, or chocolate-covered macadamia nuts. Give yourself a treat now and then. It's not going to kill you. If you don't indulge occasionally, you set yourself up for failure.

I follow a once-a-week rule. One day each week, I eat whatever I want. I've earned the right to do that by being consistent the other six days. And you know what? I don't eat half as much of the taboo treats as I used to when I ate them all the time, but I enjoy them more. That's the reward for creating good habits.

> "I'm a dedicated healthy eater, but I'm not half as extreme with my diet as I am with my workouts."

The flip side of that is you have to wake up the morning after your treat and resume your healthy eating patterns. And all the while, you have to do your cardio and resistance training, and drink tons of water.

It gets easier and easier to follow the Cover Model Diet. You're going to be absolutely elated with the way it makes you feel and look and the way it pumps your workouts. And it won't be long before you prefer to eat the healthy way and never even consider getting back on the junk food highway.

It all starts with creating the habit. So come on, let's get started. You can do it.

Meals for a Cover Model Body

Here are simple, basic menus for all five of your meals. As I mentioned in the

previous chapter, I'm not strict about measuring out precise amounts of each food. Use your common sense, and perhaps the serving-size guidelines listed on Nutrition Facts labels, to determine portion sizes.

I'm not suggesting that you

eat these meals and only these meals for the rest of your life. But I urge you to follow the guidelines until they become a habit. There's enough variety in this list for you to do that.

Once you've developed the habit of eating this way, and once you've experienced some changes to your body and attitude from the combined effects of the diet and exercise programs, you can improvise. I developed my eating and workout routines through trial and error, keeping what worked for my body, discarding what didn't. I want you to do that, too. But do it only when you understand your own body well enough to make those judgments. I started with other people's ideas and eventually personalized them to make them my own. You'll do the same. Hell, maybe in 5 years I'll be reading your book, looking for new ways to freshen up my programs.

BREAKFAST

I always have fruit and coffee with my breakfast. And it goes without saying that I drink water before and after eating.

In the previous chapter, I said I want you to spread your protein across all five meals. That can be tricky since few traditional breakfast foods are protein-rich. Eggs are the exception, of course, but you aren't going to eat five in a single morning. Though it's tempting to resort to sausage or bacon, I caution you against it. Even the lower-fat versions of those foods are made with tons of salt.

Here are some dishes you can try.

Scrambled egg whites. Scramble four egg whites—but only one yolk—with any combination of tomatoes, mushrooms, spinach, onions, bell peppers, and avocados. Have this with two slices of whole wheat toast, easy on the butter (never margarine).

Hot oat bran. This may be the best breakfast food on earth: It fills you up; gives you clean, slow-burning fuel for the first half of your day; and provides a nice dose of heart-healthy fiber and about 8 grams of protein to boot. Prepare 1 to 1½ cups using low-fat or fat-free milk, which provides more protein. Add either half of a sliced banana, some strawberries, or some raisins. A little bit of brown sugar is optional.

Cold cereal. If it's high in fiber (5 grams or more per serving), and low in sugar and sodium, it's a winner. Use low-fat or fat-free milk. I actually prefer soy milk. Sprinkle raw oat bran on top to boost the fiber and protein, or add ground flaxseed

for healthy omega-3 fats. Again, you can add banana, strawberries, or raisins to sweeten it up.

Protein smoothie. This is a great breakfast choice if you're in a rush or if you just don't feel like chewing in the morning. I prefer a whey protein powder. Put the amount you want in a blender (a scoop varies from brand to brand but is usually about 20 grams of protein) with a banana and some low-fat or fat-free milk (or low-fat yogurt). Spoon in a little peanut butter for texture and healthy fat, and let 'er rip.

For variety, try frozen berries, peaches, or even papaya instead of the banana. You can add water or ice to thin it down, if you like.

MID-MORNING
OR MID-AFTERNOON SNACK

Keep this meal down to just a few hundred calories. Again, try to include protein. It will help control your appetite, along with all its other benefits. Including protein in every meal simply makes it easier to control your weight and thus get the results you want from my program.

Protein smoothie. If you want to get 30 or more grams of protein from your snacks, you can't go wrong with a smoothie here.

Apple and peanut butter. The one downside of fruit is that it isn't always filling. Not so with apples. Eat one or two of them and you know you've eaten something substantial, even though two medium-size apples add up to only about 300 calories. Two tablespoons of peanut butter adds another 200 calories, but it's so filling you'll think it's more. Put together, this is a 500-calorie snack that feels like a full meal.

Cottage cheese. This is an excellent source of protein to go with a pure carbohydrate such as an apple or banana. It's a great source of calcium, too. Go for the low-fat version. Even if you're used to whole-milk cottage cheese, you won't even notice the taste difference after a few times.

Chicken or turkey breast. Without the skin, chicken and turkey breasts are mostly protein. You can add a small green salad with an olive oil–based dressing to get some carbohydrates and fat as well.

Tuna. Forget the mayonnaise and bread. Tuna is a pure-protein snack right out of the can. Add a little celery or other finely chopped vegetables for carbs and a little more texture, if you wish. Some guys like tuna with sweet pickles, which certainly add some flavor. Watch out for the sodium, though: One little gherkin has 128 milligrams.

Meal-replacement bar. This is, in my opinion, the best way to get your mid-morning meal without stopping work. Don't go for just any old bar, though. Check the label. You want one that emphasizes protein (not carbs) and that's relatively low in sugar.

LUNCH

The lunch choices I recommend are pretty much interchangeable with the dinner options, with one difference: Here you can sneak in some potato or rice. I'd still stay away from bread or pasta, especially if you had toast at breakfast.

Broil, grill, or bake your fish or meat, but don't use sauces on it. Season it with lemon, olive oil, garlic, pepper, vinegar, or any other spice from your cabinet.

Fish with rice. This is a classic combination. Use brown rice instead of white, which is processed like crazy. And don't pile it on; I'd rather you eat more fish than rice. Chicken also goes well with rice.

Chicken breast with green salad. Fish or lean red meat can replace the chicken. Build the salad out of fresh vegetables, including dark green lettuce. Save the iceberg lettuce for dinners at your mom's house. Don't use a creamy salad dressing—that converts a healthy dish into an unhealthy one. I like balsamic vinegar and lemon juice with a teaspoon of olive oil.

Chicken breast with baked potato. The chicken should be skinless. You can substitute lean red meat, fish, or turkey. Bet you never thought you'd hear this from me, but here goes: Enjoy your potato! Actually, enjoy half of a baked potato, and enjoy it without salt or butter. Use spices instead, and a little fat-free sour cream if you must.

Meat and vegetables. Remember to choose lean cuts of meat such as strip steak or pork loin. With any meat choice (as well as the fish and chicken breast mentioned above), you can skip the rice, salad, or potato, and go with steamed or lightly sautéed vegetables. My favorites are asparagus, broccoli (or any other dark green vegetable), cauliflower, carrots, corn, beets, or tomatoes. By no means are you limited to one veggie. Another option is beans. I prefer black, red, and garbanzo beans.

DINNER

You know the rule by now: no rice, potato, pasta, or bread. This isn't a good time for fruit, either.

Keep your meat lean—that means no skin on the chicken, and none of that marbled fat in the beef. It's not that you're trying to avoid all fat in this meal. Some fat in your stomach will probably help you sleep better since it should curb whatever urge you might have to inhale a pint of Häagen-Dazs at midnight. You just want to make the fats the ones that will be the friendliest to your waistline: the omega-3 fats in fish such as salmon, and the monounsaturated fats in olive oil. You can do without the saturated fats in meat.

> *"Some fat in your stomach will probably help you sleep better since it should curb whatever urge you might have to inhale a pint of Häagen-Dazs at midnight."*

Finally, keep in mind my idea that your dinner shouldn't be any larger than your lunch. You've been eating all day, so you shouldn't be ravenously hungry as you sit down for your evening meal.

Sautéed meat and vegetables.

Choose fish, chicken breast, turkey, or lean red meat—or any combination of those. Chop the meat into small cubes or strips, then sauté it in olive oil with similar-size pieces of dark green vegetables such as asparagus, broccoli, brussels sprouts, zucchini, or bell pepper. For more flavor, include garlic, onions, and/or basil, along with pepper (no salt) and lemon juice.

Broiled or grilled meat with vegetables.

Same idea as above, except you broil or grill the meat, and pile the vegetables on the side. I prefer a big pile of spinach that's been lightly steamed with spices, garlic, and/or onion. Other good vegetables to steam or sauté in olive oil are broccoli, asparagus, brussels sprouts, or zucchini.

Meat and raw vegetables.

The protein, as usual, can be fish, lean red meat, chicken breast, or turkey; cooked by broiling, baking, or grilling. If you like that leafy feel to your salad, raw spinach leaves are perfect. In fact, they make a great salad all by themselves. Salads aren't the only way you can enjoy raw vegetables. My favorites—all of which taste great with a vinegar–lemon–olive oil dressing—are corn right off the cob, carrots, cucumbers, tomatoes, and broccoli.

Meat and beans.

This is meat and potatoes without the potatoes. Your main course is the usual lean red meat, chicken breast, turkey, or fish. Red, black, kidney, or soybeans take the place of the spuds. It's best to buy fresh or dried beans and prepare them yourself. If you get the beans out of a can, make sure no salt, fat, or preservatives have been added. You can broil, grill, or bake the meat, and either serve it separately or cube it and mix it with the beans.

IF YOU ABSOLUTELY MUST SNACK AT NIGHT . . .

I like a type of soybean called edamame. Until recently, I came across them only at sushi restaurants, but now I find them at specialty grocery stores. They're my favorite indulgence on those rare nights when I munch away in front of the TV. Boil a whole bunch of the pods, and pop them open one by one. A little lemon juice is all you need to put on them—or not even that.

When only something sweet will do, I pop some grapes that I keep in the freezer. I'm telling you, they taste like candy. They're not something you want to eat every night, but they sure beat ice cream.

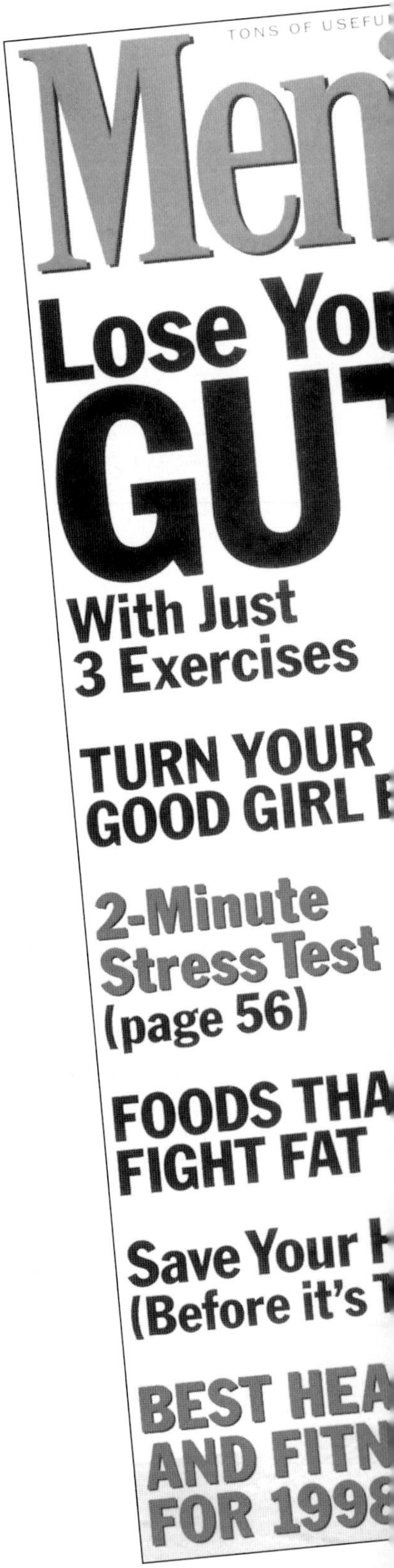

Men'

Lose You

GU

**With Just
3 Exercises**

**TURN YOUR
GOOD GIRL E**

**2-Minute
Stress Test
(page 56)**

**FOODS THA
FIGHT FAT**

**Save Your H
(Before it's T**

**BEST HEA
AND FITN
FOR 1998**

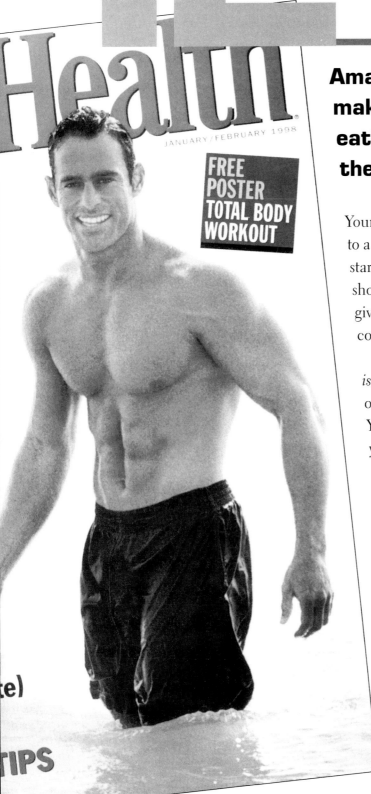

JANUARY/FEBRUARY 1998

FREE POSTER TOTAL BODY WORKOUT

Amazing things happen when you make exercise and healthy eating a habit. Have you noticed the transformation yet?

Your pants fit better. That spare tire has been reduced to a training wheel. Those garter-snake arms are starting to look more like pythons. Your back and shoulders are broadening even as your waist shrinks, giving a triumphant V shape to a torso that once could've been described as The Story of O.

Maybe it's happening fast, maybe it isn't. But it *is* happening. Even if you can't tell, you can bet others do. They've probably told you so by now. You're lean, you're buff, you're yolked . . . and if you aren't, it's at least evident that you're heading in that direction.

You're a new man on the inside, too, overflowing with energy, confidence, optimism. Clean living does that to a guy. It's happened to every guy who's ever stuck with a diet-and-exercise program persistently enough to make it a true habit. And it will happen for you, too, if it hasn't already.

Full Speed Ahead

The best is yet to come. Something even more amazing happens when you stick with a program like this for a long time—years, rather than weeks or months. It goes beyond your improved appearance and your enhanced confidence. The world around you starts coming together in your favor. The breaks go your way more often. The world starts to seem like a different place, a planet of possibilities, a place where you can hold your own, compete, win.

I started working out seriously in high school, when knee problems shot down my soccer career and kept me on crutches for half of my senior year. Barely a year later, I was offered an athletic scholarship at a major college in a sport I'd hardly played. When more injuries plagued me, I worked out even harder and soon got invited to play my second-best sport professionally.

My modeling career happened almost by accident—if you read the opening chapters of this book, you know how seriously I took the idea of getting my picture taken wearing other people's clothes. But after my back surgery, and after rededicating myself to clean living and an even higher level of fitness, modeling led me to opportunities I'd never contemplated. I not only landed on the cover of *Men's Health* magazine a record number of times but also got work as an actor and TV personality. And I became a husband and father.

Your rewards will almost certainly be different than mine, as they should be. (How many cover models does the world need, anyway?) But whatever they are, you've earned them. You deserve them.

From Habit to Hobby

The origin of all the good things that have happened for me is the habit—the practice of exercising hard, eating right, living clean. I hope you have the habit by now, and that you didn't just keep reading ahead before trying the program. But whether you have it or just want it, I want to plant this idea in your head:

Never forget that the habit is a baseline. It's the minimum you have to do to maintain your health-and-fitness foundation. You can't settle for that foundation any more than you would tell contractors to stop building your dream house after they'd successfully laid a concrete slab. You need to look for ways to add to that foundation.

Establishing a habit is by far the most important step in getting what you want from a healthy life. But it's the next step—turning your habit into a hobby—that brings the most spectacular, life-altering results. I've been talking up the habit throughout this book, and I'm not going to backpedal now. I do, however, want to explain the difference between habit and hobby.

A habit, like brushing your teeth or getting your kids ready for school, is a necessary, normal part of your life. It's automatic, a duty and a responsibility, something you do without thinking too much about it.

A hobby, on the other hand, is something you look forward to spending time on. You want to learn more. You go online to read about it and exchange information with others who share your interest. You subscribe to magazines on the topic, read books, go out of your way to absorb more and meet other people like you.

A habit you do. A hobby you look forward to doing.

I can't wait to work out each day. Sometimes I wake up and do my cardio before I even brush my teeth. And as I mentioned before, I hate to take a day off. The concept of a day without exercise just doesn't sit right with me. Also, I usually pick the hardest option if I have a choice between, say, an exercise bike and The Hill.

Some people would call this compulsive or addictive. They're wrong. I do it because I love it. I love the challenge. I love the results. I love what I learn about myself and my potential.

Most important, the way I pursue my exercise hobby doesn't keep me from getting on with the rest of my life. On the contrary, it helps me do everything else better.

Friends Don't Let Friends Get out of Shape

One of the best things you can do for your fitness program is get a support system in place. If a family member or buddy shares your goals, you'll have an easier time establishing the habit and then turning it into a hobby.

So if you like to work out with your buddies, go for it. A lot of guys find they can feed off each other's energy and get better workouts. I prefer to exercise alone, but I still like being around guys who share the same fitness lifestyle. It gets back to the hobby thing—it's just really invigorating to talk about things you're into. The enthusiasm is catching. When you mention some new restaurant where they grill fish and serve it with green beans instead of rice, it's great to be around people who say, "Hey, let's check it out," instead of, "Don't they serve pizza?"

And you learn a lot from other people. I'm very open-minded about how to do things in the gym, and I'm always scrutinizing other people's techniques. I even watch animals. Pay attention to a cat sometime—you'll learn some things about movement.

A lot of the Cover Model Workout is synthesized and modified from my observations of others, as well as my personal experience. So keep your eyes open in the gym. Some of those other guys may be revealing secrets you can use.

Family: Friends or Foes?

Even if you don't have or want a workout partner, at least try to get those closest to you to cheer you on instead of telling you how crazy you are. Easier said than done, right? When your boss needs you to work overtime to keep the company afloat, or your wife needs more help at home, or your kid needs help with his homework, it's hard to find cheerleaders. You probably think I can't relate to all this, but I can. I mean, I can't go to the gym every time I get the urge. I have work obligations. I have a wife and son who sometimes need me more than I need to pump blood into my muscles. And I do this for a living!

The key, I think, is to view your other responsibilities as a way to make workouts more focused and efficient. If Lisa tells me I have only a half-hour to work out because we have to do this or that, I have to find some way to make those 30 minutes as productive as 2 hours at the gym. That usually means sprints on the street outside the house.

As I'm writing this, my son, Blaze, is not quite 3 years old. When it's one of my days to take care of him, I don't even consider skipping my workout. I strap him into his stroller and push him up The Hill. Or I take him with me to The Stairs, skipping my pushups and pullups, and instead concentrating on taking the steps

"If a family member or buddy shares your goals, you'll have an easier time establishing the habit."

two at a time with 40 pounds of toddler resistance on my shoulders. Blaze loves it, and for me the workout has a double benefit: Not only is it a killer but it makes my child-free workouts on The Stairs seem easy by comparison.

The dinner table is another place where you need your family on your side (but not on your back). As you get into the Cover Model Diet, you change a lot of eating habits—not just what you eat but also how much and when. The best-case scenario is that the rest of the household gets with the program and eats healthy right along with you. If that's not realistic, it's up to you to explain your diet and create a routine that lets everybody eat the way they want without disrupting family unity.

This gets really hard at extended-family gatherings, where a food-pushing aunt or in-law takes it personally if you don't stuff yourself with her sausage and pasta. My advice is to not fight it. Spare her feelings and consider the meal a special treat. Just find a way to drink tons of water, and make sure you get back on track the next day.

If these get-togethers are weekly occasions, you need to take some defensive action. Open your mouth and explain what you're trying to do for yourself with healthy eating and exercise. Don't be sanctimonious and imply that you're going to fitness heaven while they're condemned to a hell of clogged arteries and insulin resistance. Make it clear that this a choice you felt that you had to make, but that you don't expect the rest of the family to change. All you ask is for them to respect your choices. They may go even further and try to accommodate your new diet. You can't expect that, but it could happen, if you approach your relatives the right way.

Steal This Workout

When you fit in a workout even though all the odds are against you, you've stolen one. Say you don't have any exercise scheduled but you find yourself with time to kill and decide to lace up your shoes and do 20 minutes of sprints anyway. That's stealing one. When it's Saturday night at the brew pub and you have a chicken breast, a pitcher of water, and one or two beers while your buddies devour mountains of spaghetti and drain the beer vats, you've robbed one right out from under their garlicky noses.

There are a million ways to steal a workout. Use a negative fitness experience as motivation to do something extra. Dinner party tonight? Do a half-hour lifting circuit before your shower. The extra cardiovascular and strength work will offset the looming calorie fest. Plus, you jump-start your metabolism to minimize the damage.

I do a lot of stealing on modeling days. The truth is, not many people at photo shoots are in good shape. Sometimes I'm the only one who is. The lunches are almost always out of control. They're also long since photographers don't like to shoot when the sun is high. So when the rest of the gang is feasting at the buffet table, I take off and bust an incredible workout.

Or say I arrive at a hotel with no time to hit the health spa. Instead of tipping the bellboy, I walk up the stairwell to the top floor, bags and all. Then I take the elevator down and go back up the stairs again. I've stolen one before I've even seen my room.

You should always be looking for ways to steal a workout. Things you normally hate doing can become a chance to burn a few more calories. For example, helping somebody move is a great opportunity to steal one. (And having visibly strong muscles is like having a pickup truck: Anybody who's moving will ask for your help.) Carrying all that furniture around is like circuit training—cardio and resistance training combined. And the more stairs you have to climb, the better.

I remember one day when I figured I'd have to blow off my usual workout because I had to renew my driver's license before taking off for a long flight. Now, what's a bigger drag than standing in line at the Department of Motor Vehicles? But instead of complaining (too much, anyway), I asked myself how I could steal a workout out of this. I ended up running to the DMV, getting my license, then running back.

Here's the most satisfying way to steal one: Do something you know hardly anybody else will do. That automatically puts you ahead of the pack. That's why I love to wake up and see that it's raining hard outside. There's no rule against working out in the rain, but I know The Stairs will be empty. Empty, that is, until I get there to steal one.

Every time you steal a workout, it's a bonus. It's more calories burned, more muscle built, more time tacked onto your life. Steal a few

> "You should always be looking for ways to steal a workout."

every week and by the time a year is up, you'll have deposited wads of cold, hard fitness in your body's bank.

You'll be surprised how many times you can steal one if your goal is doing as much exercise as possible, instead of as little as you can get away with. In other words, you can steal a lot if you really want to.

Taking the Show on the Road

Any wine aficionado or golf nut looks at travel as a chance to expand his hobby's horizons: to taste new wine, play an exotic course, meet others who share his passion. Travel can present the same range of opportunities to a fitness enthusiast.

I do plenty of business traveling, and 9 times out of 10 I come back from a trip in better shape than when I left. I find a way to get my work in, and often I find a way to do better work.

If I have an early flight out, for example, I set the alarm for 3:30 A.M. and do the hardest workout I can do in the least amount of time. I'll find myself at The Stairs at 4:00 in the morning—just me and the raccoons. And when I'm done, I'm already way ahead of the game. My workout is in, my metabolism is primed to handle any calories that get thrown at me on the trip, and I'm already drinking a ton of water to smooth out the effects of the flight.

I don't touch the food they serve on the plane. It's loaded with preservatives and sodium, and usually too much saturated fat. True, it's hard to resist sometimes—I'm hungry, it smells good,

and what else is there to do on a plane anyway? But I arm myself with a meal-replacement bar, maybe some healthy snack I've packed, and double my usual water.

Try my flight plan the next time you go airborne. When you get off a plane knowing you're the only one who didn't open the complimentary peanuts, you'll feel empowered. You'll have a victory under your belt and the momentum to carry it through for the rest of your time on the road.

> "When you get off a plane knowing you're the only one who didn't open the complimentary peanuts, you'll feel empowered."

I try to get in a workout at the hotel before I even unpack my bags. When you check in, look at it as arriving at a gym instead of a hotel. The equipment in the hotel's fitness room will probably be different from what you're used to. If it's different in a good way, you'll get to play around with some new machines and try some new exercises. If it's interesting in a bad way— the norm, unfortunately—ask the hotel concierge for names of gyms where you can work out on a day pass. Many hotels have arrangements with local health clubs that will let you work out for free or at a discounted day rate. That can be even more fun, especially if the gym is bigger and better-equipped than your hometown club.

Another alternative is to worry about the gym later and get in a cardio workout right off. A quick run or brisk walk can give you a good idea of your options for meals and even nightlife.

You may end up getting more exercise on a travel day than you normally get when you don't travel. And believe me, you'll notice the differ-

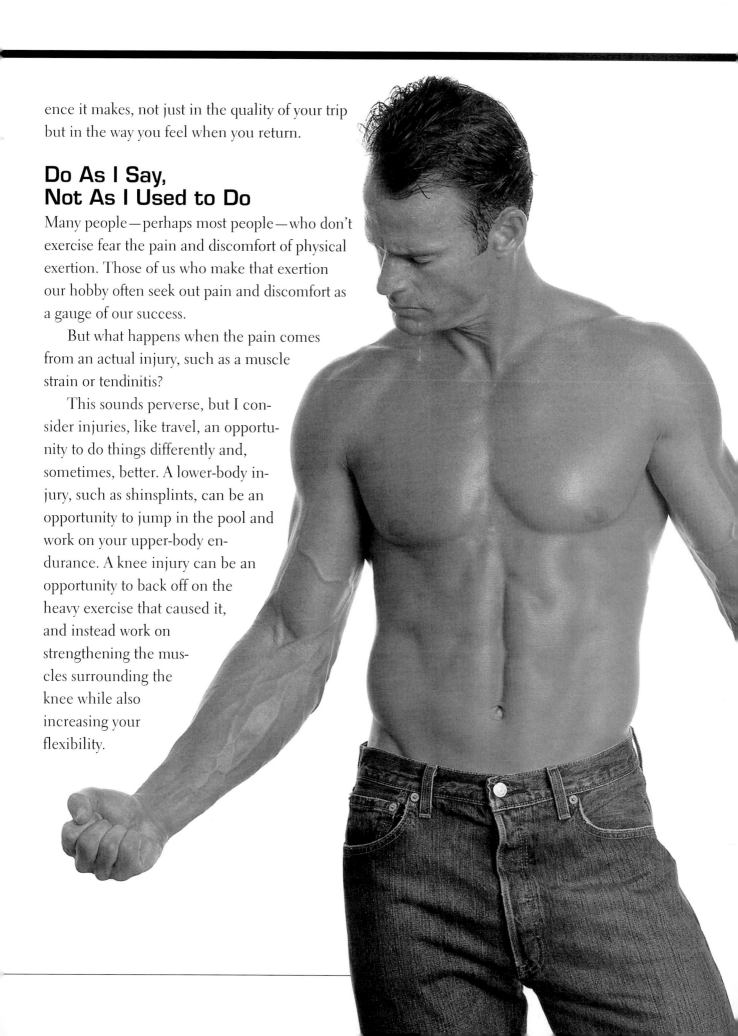

ence it makes, not just in the quality of your trip but in the way you feel when you return.

Do As I Say,
Not As I Used to Do

Many people—perhaps most people—who don't exercise fear the pain and discomfort of physical exertion. Those of us who make that exertion our hobby often seek out pain and discomfort as a gauge of our success.

But what happens when the pain comes from an actual injury, such as a muscle strain or tendinitis?

This sounds perverse, but I consider injuries, like travel, an opportunity to do things differently and, sometimes, better. A lower-body injury, such as shinsplints, can be an opportunity to jump in the pool and work on your upper-body endurance. A knee injury can be an opportunity to back off on the heavy exercise that caused it, and instead work on strengthening the muscles surrounding the knee while also increasing your flexibility.

Elbow tendinitis? It's a sign that you're over-doing something. And if you're overdoing something, you're almost certainly neglecting something else. So you figure out what those somethings are and you fix the problems.

You may end up doing more exercise while rehabilitating an injury and trying to prevent a recurrence. The net effect: You know more about your body, and you're even more dedicated to improving its condition.

That said, I have to admit I'm not exactly the poster child for injury recognition and smart rehabilitation. If I'd paid enough attention to what my body was telling me, I would have had rotator cuff surgery 5 years earlier and had my back bolted together a decade before I finally did. My instincts have always been to eat the pain. My mantra: Pain is just weakness leaving your body.

Part of me even likes pain. Sometimes I hit the gym and just beat myself up physically so that the next day I'll wake up so sore I can feel the webbing in my toes. I know it sounds weird, but it's kind of a cool feeling—like I've left the party with a really nice parting gift.

You don't need to go to that extreme. In fact, you'll be a lot better off if you don't. Still, everyone who works out hard, who challenges himself to do better, will eventually get hurt. In theory, it's easy to distinguish between the normal soreness that accompanies hard exercise and a genuine injury. In reality, you have to suffer a few injuries before you get the hang of making the distinction, and even then you often

"I consider injuries opportunities to do things differently and, sometimes, better."

have to fight off the instinct to just keep pushing in hopes the injury heals on its own.

Sometimes, a twinge hurts like hell for a few seconds, and then quits as suddenly as it began, allowing you to finish your workout without any repercussions. Other times, a subtle ache can be the first sign of an overuse injury, and working through it will only make it worse.

Here's how you can diagnose yourself in the weight room: Grab a weight that's a lot lighter than you'd normally use for that exercise. See if you can do a set of the exercise, using a full range of motion. If you can do that without discomfort, rest for a minute, and perhaps stretch the muscles in question. Then try another set. Most of the time after you feel a twinge, you'll be pain-free after a couple of light-weight sets. If the discomfort persists, stop, and spend the rest of your workout time on exercises that don't affect the injured area.

Test the area again the next week. Or, if you're convinced that you're truly injured, see a doctor.

Another useful diagnostic tool is the two-workout test. If a muscle or joint hurts in the same place two workouts in a row, it's injured. Come up with a plan for resting, rehabilitating, and preventing a recurrence.

From Hobby to Career

My body has always been my meal ticket. As my beach volleyball career unfolded, it was already clear that whatever the next chapter of my life was to be, my body would be a big part of it.

That was one of the motivating forces that got me to the gym every day in those otherwise unrestrained times.

In volleyball, my performance counted, not my appearance. So it wasn't really until I started doing body modeling for *Men's Health* that I actually got paid for the way I looked. And I have to tell you, it's always felt a little strange that people would pay me to stand there and let them photograph me. It's flattering, and I love doing it, but it's weird to think that my job is to stay in shape. My hobby had officially become a career.

The kind of shape you're in is a huge factor in any kind of modeling. When I first started doing fashion stuff, I was too big, at 220 pounds, and thick, with a 19½-inch neck. It was made pretty clear to me that if I wanted to work, I'd have to trim down—even though I had a single-digit body-fat percentage. There wasn't much more I could lose unless I started chopping off body parts.

But the fashion industry figures that men who've muscled up in a way that makes them look really big aren't going to look right in clothes. It's the Arnold Schwarzenegger syndrome: Here's a guy with an awesome body who just never looks natural in a suit. I had to adjust my training regimen to go for a hard, lean look—plenty of muscle, less emphasis on size. So even back in my fashion days, professional factors influenced my workouts.

With the kind of shots I do for *Men's Health*, training is everything. I still don't go for too much size, especially since I tend to photograph big. I'm 6 foot 2, and people assume from the

> *"What you look like at your peak can improve from year to year."*

covers that I weigh about 220 pounds. But I'm rarely over 200.

There's nothing like shirtless magazine-cover work to motivate you to get into shape. Literally millions of people are going to see me. One image might appear on 22 covers, in 30 countries. But what really fuels my workouts is the competition to get on the cover in the first place. All those covers under my belt don't guarantee that the next one will be mine. And even when the magazine calls me, I'm still not necessarily a shoe-in. *Men's Health* may shoot three or four models for a cover and go with the one who works best.

So the rivalries can get pretty heated. As you know by now, that's the kind of challenge that I live for. By the time you read this, I'll be 40, making me one of the oldest guys vying for the kind of work I do. So even if I weren't naturally inclined to work harder than the next guy, I'd have to anyway, just to stay in business. Some of the younger guys think they have me beat just by showing up. They may follow a stricter diet than I do (and some of them may get a little extra help that they'll never fess up to), but nobody works harder than me. That's something I can pretty much guarantee.

Tricks of the Trade

When it's almost time to shoot a cover, I adjust my diet and exercise to achieve a peak. Every guy has moments in his life when he wants to be in peak condition, such as when the girl who dumped him in high school says she'll be in town in 2 weeks and wants to get together.

Whatever your peak moments are, the habit—the fitness foundation—makes the peaks possible. You have a baseline level of fitness, which translates to a baseline appearance. That puts you near your peak most of the time, and puts you in position to take it up a level when circumstances demand.

What you look like at your peak can improve from year to year. That's because your baseline can improve from one year to the next, so your baseline next year might be what your peak looks like now. When I talk about a peak, I mean a condition that's about 10 percent better than what you look like at your current baseline, not an appearance that's the absolute best you can ever attain. I want you to understand how relative all this is, and how hard work produces continual rewards year after year.

When I'm peaking for a cover, I try to get my weight down to the low 190s. To do that, I up my protein, cut back on my carbohydrates, and keep my fats pretty much the same. I still eat nuts (unsalted, of course), avocados, olive oil, and fatty fish. But I cut down my overall calorie intake. I also enact a zero-tolerance policy for sugar, and I pretty much eliminate high-glycemic carbohydrates (potatoes, pasta, rice, and bread).

At the same time, I increase the intensity of my workouts. That can mean lifting heavier weights with fewer repetitions. For me, it also means a lot of sprinting, and maybe running The Stairs a few times instead of walking up them 10 times.

Another secret for getting cover ready—or peaking for any reason—is to do workouts you don't normally do. For 2 or 3 days before a shoot, I jump in the pool to do the water routines that I trot out only on select occasions. That gets my whole body tingling. My back blows up and my shoulders pop. And it all happens almost instantly.

The final touch comes in the last 24 hours before the photo session. After 2 weeks of carbohydrate depletion, I pop a potato in the oven and eat half of it the night before the shoot. Then I eat the other half the next morning.

That does exactly what I've been begging you to avoid at all other times: It causes a sugar rush. The sugar soaks up the water in the tissues between my muscles and outer skin so my muscles are visibly pumped. I prolong the effect by popping frozen grapes during the shoot itself, which also gets the veins popping.

My way: Learn stupid model tricks. As long as I'm revealing the tricks of the trade, let me clue you in on some of the little things you can do to please the camera. Even if you never model for any magazine, you're going to get your picture taken from time to time, like it or not. And who doesn't want to look better in a picture that, in theory, is going to be around long after you're gone?

The first thing you go for, if you have any control over it, is to get the shot taken outdoors in the daytime. The heat from natural sunshine brings out your vascularity. You show more definition. If you're going to smile, make some noise when you do it. Laughing works best. Just keep your chin down and chuckle out loud. Think about it. When you smile silently for the camera, it almost always looks cheesy and contrived. But a smile with sound is a natural smile. Besides, you exhale when you laugh, so your stomach tightens and your torso looks great.

Don't stand square to the camera, with your body facing it straight on. You'll look square. Stand at a three-quarter angle. Or offset your shoulders a bit so one is closer to the camera than the other. Try looking slightly away from the camera and see how that positioning comes out. You can also experiment with looking down a bit.

The Road to Opportunity

When you're working your tail off at the gym or dodging raccoons on The Stairs at 4:00 in the morning, you sometimes need to remind yourself of the rewards that come with your efforts. As I've tried to make clear, the main reward of exercise is in doing it. It makes you healthier. Anything else is gravy.

Still, I'd always figured there'd be more of a payoff to my hard work than cover modeling. The honor of being the face of the *Men's Health* brand is something I cherish and will always carry with me. But in the big picture, I figured there'd be more. And I'm hungry for it.

I still don't know what "more" will include. But I've had some intriguing hints. Dan Rather's crew from the TV newsmagazine *48 Hours* followed me around for a few days while I was doing a cover shoot. My Web site, AskOwen.com, went up when the show aired and got 48,000 hits the first day.

Later, the entertainment-news show *Extra!* did a segment on a *Men's Health* shoot, featuring four cover models. I hit them with my press kit and a pitch to take me on as their fitness guy. I threw a well-baited hook out there, and they nibbled. I got a meeting and went to work on them in my own fashion, pointing at each one of the assembled execs, male and female. "You, you want to lose that gut? I'll show you the way. You, want to trim those thighs? Here's how." And so on around the room, boom boom boom.

Next thing I knew, they were asking me to do a segment on how to get washboard abs. I've been a semiregular *Extra!* fitness correspondent ever since, logging dozens of appearances.

Now that I've gotten a taste of TV, I'm seeking out more opportunities. My pet project is a health, fitness, and wellness show for the whole family. I'd tell a mom and dad how to get themselves back into shape while they help their teenager stay healthy and feed their little one the best after-school snacks. I think it's a show the world needs, and I still plan to do it.

> "My pet project is a health, fitness, and wellness show for the whole family. . . . I think it's a show the world needs, and I still plan to do it."

But some tantalizing possibilities have arisen while I've been trying to get it off the ground. One day in 2001, I was pitching the idea to some TV execs at the St. Regis Hotel in Los Angeles. One of the gentlemen explained that he was only an observer. I didn't hear another word out of him the entire meeting. When it was over, I gave him my card. He didn't give me his.

Two weeks later, my phone rang and a deep, distinguished voice asked for me by name. I swear I thought it was the IRS. But it was Neil Russell, the observer from that meeting, who turned out to be the creator of a proposed new television series called *Spartacus*, inspired by the success of the movie *Gladiator*. He wanted to warn me that MGM would be tracking me down because they were interested in having me play the lead. "If it's something you're not interested in," he said, "figure out a creative way to say no."

Saying no, creatively or otherwise, wasn't exactly on my mind.

The casting director contacted me and set up a meeting. Then he canceled it. He scheduled another meeting and canceled that one too. This is the way things work in Hollywood. It's expected. So I did what was expected of me. I called and told him that I was a busy man with a heavy traveling schedule, and that I didn't have time to fool around. Get me in a room, one time, with everybody who needs to be there. Then make a decision. Let's do it.

MGM sent me two scenes and set up a meeting for me to read them. It was an audition, and it wasn't canceled.

Neil Russell had written the scenes I was to read, and he gave me some advice about delivering the lines: Hold nothing back. Don't leave the room wishing I'd done something that I hadn't. I had his permission to do everything but tear the people's heads off.

I'd done some television acting, the kind a young, well-built guy in L.A. can pick up with a little effort. Six episodes of *Pacific Blue*. One *Suddenly Susan*. Some soap work. Still, acting doesn't come to me as naturally as staying physically fit does. So Neil's help was greatly needed. I also had assistance from another source: my wife. Rehearsing with Lisa taught me to listen. And listening is the key to acting, as far as I'm concerned. The trick is to respond to a line as though you were hearing it for the first time, not the thousandth, which is more likely the case. You can do that only by really listening to it.

So there I was, walking through the hallowed halls of MGM, past more Oscars than I knew existed. When I was a kid on the beach in Hawaii, I tried to match the footsteps my big brothers made hopping in the sand. Now I was following in the footsteps of Kirk Douglas and Russell Crowe. No pressure there.

I took Neil Russell's advice to heart. Long story short, I ended up spitting at the guy feeding me my lines. I shed tears. I got so intense my lips shook. And I left the room feeling pretty good. I got the part.

A Future without Limits Awaits You

I've told you my whole Spartacus story for a reason—and it's not to feed my ego. Heck, I don't even know if the series will ever air, just as I don't know if I'll still be on *Extra!* next season. My point is this: I wasn't considered for the gladiator role because somebody mistook me for Robert De Niro. I was considered as a direct result of my physical condition.

Neil Russell was clear about that when he called 20 minutes after the MGM meeting to congratulate me. It turned out the project had been in development for a couple of years, and they'd had no luck finding a guy in his thirties who they felt could stay in top shape for 9 months out of the year. The shooting was planned for Malta and Australia, and TV people know that an actor who looks right for the part at the outset tends to soften up under grueling conditions on the other side of the world. You can't have a hero like Spartacus played by a guy with flabby pecs. After listening to me for an hour at that meeting, Neil knew that I wouldn't let my

physique deteriorate, no matter how exhausting the work turned out to be.

I got the part because of those cold, foggy mornings at The Stairs; those hot, sweaty afternoons on The Hill; those endless hours in the weight room. The twin pillars of fitness, consistency and discipline, put me in position for this opportunity. I've been preaching this since chapter 1, but I can't resist saying it one more time: They work.

They probably won't work for you the same way they worked for me. I don't imagine too many of you aspire to a life in front of the camera. But I don't think I'm being naive when I say that the lessons you learn by getting and staying fit translate to all other pursuits. What aspects of life aren't improved with consistency and discipline? Your employer will have more confidence in you when you follow through and stick with a project until it's finished. Women will take you more seriously when you establish that you're somebody who strives for self-improvement, who tries every day to get better.

There's another way that the fitness lessons I've been teaching you paid off for me. Going for a lead television role at this stage of my life presented a huge challenge. Most of the actors you see on TV or in the movies have been developing their skill since they were children. The fact that I hadn't even attempted it until my thirties could've deterred me, but it didn't. I took it as yet another challenge and ran with it. I went after it with the same fitness-inspired confidence that landed me an athletic career in a sport I'd hardly ever played, and then a modeling career that I knew next to nothing about going in.

Find motivation, be persistent, and let adversity be a reason to do more instead of less. Those are the three major lessons of the Cover Model Workout. They've served me every step of the way. My life is proof that they work. They'll work for you in ways you can't even conceive of in advance.

It's Never Too Late

I consider myself a late bloomer. Although I was genetically blessed with athletic skills that blossomed at an early age, in other ways I was way behind other kids. I mean, I had some of my baby teeth until I was 18. I had to have them yanked so the permanent teeth could grow in. I got my silver braces put on well after most people get theirs off. I didn't get my driver's license until I was 19 (which may have had something to with my "borrowing" my mom's car at age 15 and returning it with no fewer than five tickets). I even wet the bed long after kids usually stop, but I'll spare you that story.

My life kept on that way. I was late on everything. I didn't seriously take up my collegiate sport until I was already in college. I got discov-

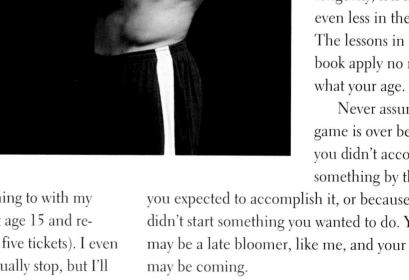

ered as a model at age 29, the twilight of many modeling careers. And now, pushing 40, I'm breaking into television.

The lesson is clear: It's never too late to find your niche, to begin something that feels right to you. We're living in times when women in their nineties are taking up weight training for the first time. The other day I heard about a man in his eighties suing to get accepted to law school. Age doesn't matter now, and as science advances our knowledge of health, fitness, and longevity, it'll matter even less in the future. The lessons in this book apply no matter what your age.

Never assume the game is over because you didn't accomplish something by the age you expected to accomplish it, or because you didn't start something you wanted to do. You may be a late bloomer, like me, and your day may be coming.

Never, Ever Give Up

Sometimes in pickup basketball I see guys walking off the court with their team down by three or four baskets and only 10 to 15 seconds left. I ask myself whether I'd want my son to see me doing that. The answer is no. I want him to see me chasing the ball like a crazy person until the clock expires.

Never give up on anything, especially your health. There are going to be times when you get frustrated with your workouts. You're going to be tempted to say to hell with it. But do me a favor. Don't quit. Ever.

I've lived long enough to know that good things come when you least expect them. And some of the best things show up when the clock is running down in overtime. You may be 10 pounds away from an agent handing you his card. You may meet your soul mate at the gym tomorrow. You never know what's around the corner.

"Never give up on anything, especially your health."

Persistence and discipline always pay off. I'm living proof of that. So please keep at it. Make the Cover Model Workout a permanent part of your life. You never know what can happen.

REACHING YOUR PEAK

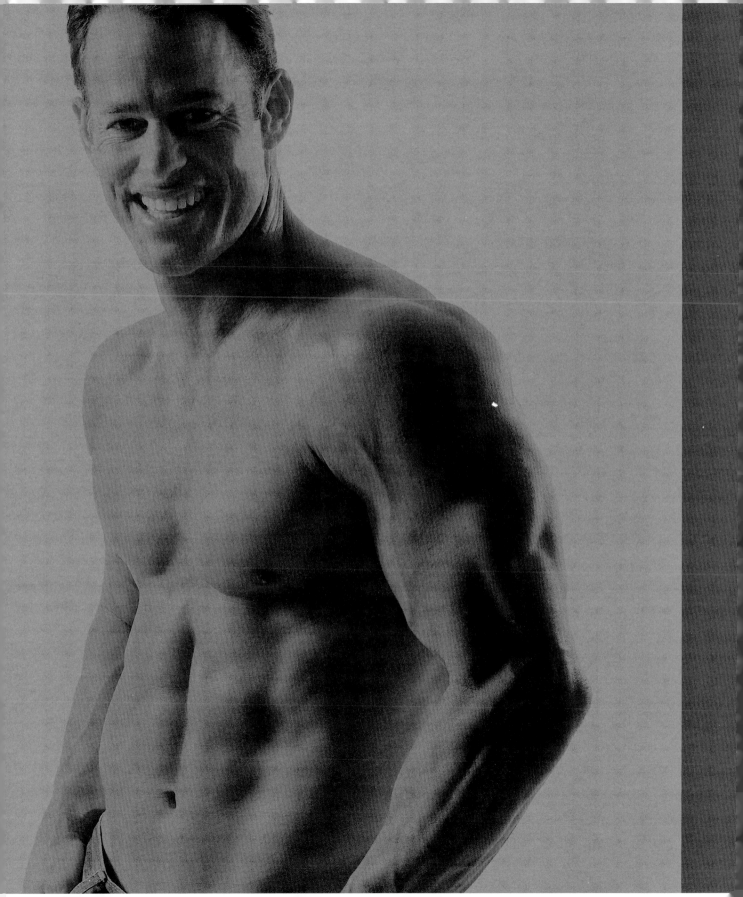

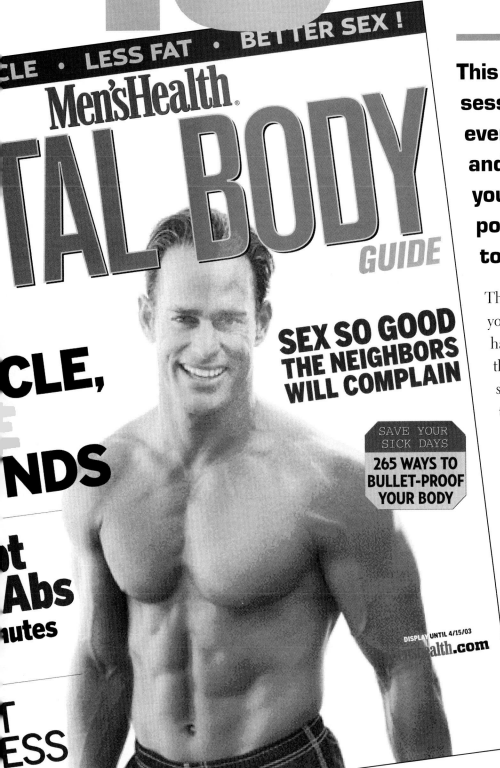

This 14-day pit session will get you even more ripped and buffed when you absolutely, positively have to look your best.

There are times in life when your mission is clear: You have to get yourself into over-the-top, stratosphere-level shape. And you have to get there quick. I'm going to show you how to do it in just 14 days.

Why is it urgent to peak out sometimes? There are lots of possible reasons.

Your 10- or 20-year high school reunion is coming up, and you want to impress the hell out of everybody you knew in your wonder years.

Your ex is cruising back into town, and

you want her to regret for the rest of her life that she dumped you.

A big Mexico weekend is planned, and this time you're going to get your share of the action.

You're starting a new job. You're going to tour Europe. You're getting married. You got a surprise invite to an A-list party. You've realized that you're out of shape, and you want to look great now. You've been assigned to liberate hostages in the jungles of Borneo.

Whatever it is, it motivates you to take your training to the next level. It knocks you into peak mode.

For me, it's a cover gig.

When I get a call from *Men's Health*, it's never an appointment I put on my calendar for later in the year. I have to be ready for that shoot ASAP. I'm lucky if I get 2 weeks' notice.

And make no mistake about it: I use that time to tweak my body into better shape, no matter how diligent I've been about my program up to then. I don't have a choice. You're only as good as your last cover, and if I'm just a speck below perfect, I'm toast.

So I use those 2 weeks to put my conditioning into overdrive. I turn myself into one big fat-burning, muscle-building organism. I literally eat and sleep fitness. My wife will attest that I'm not the most fun person to be around for those 14 days. But come C Day (cover day), I am at my absolute best.

And you can be, too. Using my own routines as a guide, I've put together for you a 14-day pro-

> "I've put together for you a 14-day program that tells you exactly what to do to reach your physical peak right when you need to the most."

gram that tells you exactly what to do to reach your physical peak right when you need to the most. I'll take you through the paces, almost hour by hour. I'll tell you specifically what to eat, what to lift, and what to do for cardio.

It's a challenge, no doubt about it. But if you promise to stick with it and follow my instructions, I promise that you'll be stunned at how great you look and feel at the end.

Remember one thing: This is a crash course, an emergency procedure. It is *not* something you can or should keep up year-round. When the 2-Week Tweak has done its job, put it aside. Your wife or girlfriend(s) will welcome you back.

Before we dive into the actual program, let me be more specific about what makes this 2-Week Tweak unique. Essentially, it's a three-pronged approach consisting of extra cardio, more intense strength training, and a strict diet. Let's take a quick look at those three elements.

Daily Cardio

You're going to do cardio every day, and you're going to do it early. The first thing that happens when you wake up (after coffee, of course) is 30 to 40 minutes of cardio at a challenging pace, or 20 minutes of sprinting. I'll let you know which to do as I give you each day's instructions, but the early start isn't optional. I want your metabolism in high gear all day long, and sunrise cardio work is the way to crank it up there.

The goal is to minimize your body fat as you

add muscle. Even if you're not overweight, improving your ratio of lean body mass to body fat is a healthy thing to do. And it's an improvement that shows. In this case, it shows *quickly*.

Intense Strength Training

"Intense" means heavier weight loads with (usually) fewer repetitions. I'll do my part to raise the intensity by prescribing your number of sets and reps. It's your job to jack up your poundages (without sacrificing good form) and to minimize your rest between sets.

The sessions (always in the P.M.) will usually be shorter than you may be used to, but with a handful of exceptions, you'll do weight work every day. You're going to be sore as hell a lot of the time, but you're also going to end up more awesomely shredded than you've ever imagined.

Strict Diet

This may be the toughest aspect of the Tweak. Your diet for these 2 weeks will be based on the same principles as the regular Cover Model Diet, but those principles will be applied with ruthless rigor. I'd never expect you to maintain these eating habits for more than 2 weeks. In fact, I don't want you to. It wouldn't be healthy in the long run. But trust me, if you follow my instructions, you'll be blown away by the results.

Basically, your overall calories will be down, your protein intake will be up, you'll eat about the same amount of fat, and your carbohydrates will be relegated to a bit role.

"Your diet for these 2 weeks will be based on the same principles as the regular Cover Model Workout, but those principles will be applied with ruthless rigor."

Meal size. Throughout this book, I've promoted the virtues of scattering five small meals over the day rather than eating two or three big ones. Now I'm going to insist you do this.

Protein. You'll aim for about a gram of protein per pound of body weight. It will come from plenty of chicken, fish, turkey, lean red meat, egg whites, protein bars, and smoothies made with protein powder. It will *not* come from dairy products, such as milk, cheese, or yogurt. They're on hold for 2 weeks.

Dietary fat. There's no need to reduce here, assuming you're used to healthy levels of dietary fat. The fat you'll get will be from olive or flaxseed oil, avocado, natural peanut butter, and meat. It will help you feel satisfied. Strictly forbidden are saturated or hydrogenated fats from the likes of butter, margarine, sauces, dressings, fat-loaded cuts of meat, chicken skin or turkey skin, mayonnaise, et cetera.

Dry carbs. Here's where you're really going to take the usual Cover Model Diet rule to extremes. In your quest to reduce your body's conversion of blood sugar to fat, you'll gradually eliminate dry carbs: pasta, potatoes, rice, and bread. You'll eat no pasta at all, no potatoes until the last 24 hours, eventually no rice (and initially only brown rice in the daytime), and no more than one piece of wheat toast in the mornings.

Vegetables. These are carbs you'll eat plenty of. Unlike dry carbs, vegetables have a low glycemic index, meaning they convert to sugar more slowly. And as you know, they're loaded with nutrients that you need whether you're tweaking or not. Plus, when you think about it, a typical meal of white or red meat and vegetables (and even brown rice at lunch for much of the program) makes for pretty good eating. Hey, my aim is to get you into peak condition, not starve you.

Sugar. For 2 weeks, a zero-tolerance policy for sugar will be in force. You'll even eat very little fruit because of the natural sugar in it. Dessert? There's no such thing during the 2-Week Tweak.

Salt. If you're used to pouring salt over everything, you're about to have an interesting experience. Salt is out for these 2 weeks.

I realize this can be a tough one. For a lot of guys, unsalted meat or vegetables are an abomination. Consider it a challenge as well as an invitation to explore the zillions of spices that are out there. If you come out of this ready to permanently cut down your salt intake, you'll have improved your health.

Alcohol. None for the duration. It's sugar, which you don't need, and it interferes with sound sleep.

Water. I've told you so many times to drink tons of water that you probably don't want to hear it anymore. Well, stand back. I'm going to tell you about a half-dozen more times a day in the pages ahead.

How to Use This Guide

First of all, relax and enjoy yourself. I've done all the thinking for you, based on what I've had to

"For 2 weeks, a zero-tolerance policy for sugar will be in force."

do to peak out when needed. All you have to do is follow the program.

To help you do that, I present the program one day at a time. After a brief preview of what's in store for each day, your exercise and meal instructions are given in order, at the time they're to be done.

Do you have to follow the schedule to the minute? I hope you do. If you need to adjust it a bit to accommodate your work or your family, go ahead. But maintain the integrity of the schedule. By that I mean keep everything in the same order, and maintain the same time between meals and mini-meals (usually 2½ hours). Always do your cardio before breakfast and your weight work in the afternoon.

Along with your workout and meal instructions, I clue you in on how to prepare the meals you'll eat for the first time on any one day. There's nothing in each day's "Kitchen Tactics" that's going to make it onto the Food Network. What you get instead is a basic, easy-to-follow how-to that will put the food on your plate without undue hassle. For this 14-day trek, there are even special instructions for your breakfast toast. Even if you're Emeril's cousin, read my recipes anyway. The instructions are specific to the requirements of the 2-Week Tweak. Some of what you think you already know may not apply.

The "Kitchen Tactics" are also useful when you're ordering your meal in a restaurant. I recommend preparing your own meals so you have control over what's in them. But if you do eat out, insist that your order adheres to the requirements I give.

After "Kitchen Tactics" come the photos that show you how to perform all the ab exercises and weight-training movements you'll do that day. The first time each exercise appears, I'll give you a written description—if it shows up again, you'll just see photos. You will already be familiar with some of the exercises from the regular Cover Model Workout. But I present them all again for two reasons. One is that there may be some subtle differences in technique. The other is that I don't want you to have to keep thumbing all over the book to find the exercise you need.

For each day, you'll also find a chart listing all that day's activities: cardio, abs, and weights. You can use this as a convenient checklist as you go through your routines, plus as a running log of your performance.

For your cardio work, the log tells you the kind of training I want you to do that day (steady pace, intervals, or sprints) and the range of minutes you should do it for. You can record the actual number of minutes you complete and (if you find it useful) what mode you used (jogging, treadmill, stationary bike, et cetera).

True to my philosophy, you won't be maniacal about your ab work. Some days you won't even do any abdominal exercises. Rest assured that the draconian diet I'm putting you on will do more to show off your six-pack than endless ab exercises. Still, abs are muscles, so we're

"No matter what your fitness level, I guarantee that if you attack this workout like the mad animal I know you are, you're going to love what you look and feel like come Day 14."

going to give them some work to do most days.

For both the ab and weight work, I give you the exercise and the number of reps you should do for each set. You write in the weight you used (when applicable) for each set and the number of reps you actually completed. That info can help you move to a higher weight or more reps when you repeat that exercise another day.

Finally, a word for beginners: If you haven't been working out at all but you still want to give the 2-Week Tweak a shot, you're my kind of human being. Be smart, though. The last thing you need is to get discouraged from taking on too much too soon. You can still do the program and reap the benefits. But make adjustments. For example, you might start off with walking instead of jogging. Or cut the 30-minute cardio sessions into two 15-minute sessions, or even three at 10 minutes each. In the weight room, keep the poundage down so you can finish the reps in all the prescribed sets—but don't cut it so far down that the movements are too easy. Concentrate on good form. And if you can't quite complete the reps of an ab exercise despite trying your best . . . hell, that's as good as a burnout set.

On the positive side, you can stick to my eating plan as well as the most experienced tweaker can.

No matter what your fitness level, I guarantee that if you attack this workout like the mad animal I know you are, you're going to love what you look and feel like come Day 14.

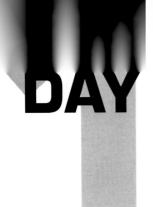

DAY 1

Dude, start your engine.
Your 2-week race to peak condition is under way.

There won't be any special pep talk from me today. I know you're already supermotivated. You're ready. I'm ready. So let's do it.

We're going to start right in with all pistons firing: cardio, abs, strength training, and focused nutrition. If you've been following the Cover Model Workout, the only really radical departure from your usual routine may be the 6:00-A.M. start. Get used to it. You absolutely need to get a lot done before breakfast, so from now on you're an early bird. If anything, you may need to set the alarm even earlier—especially if you do your cardio at a gym that you need some time to get to.

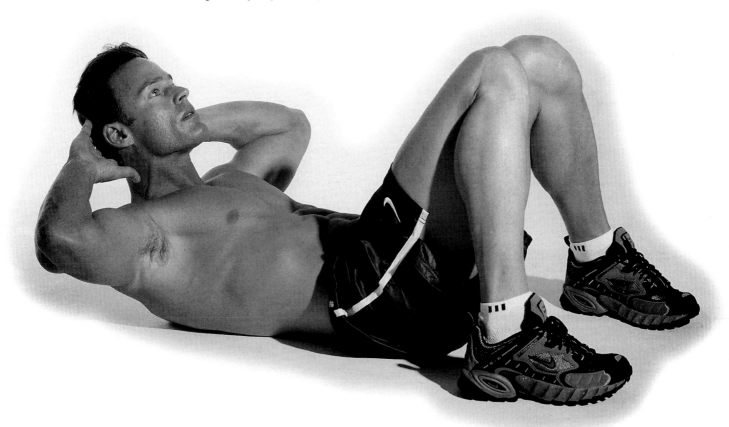

6:00 A.M.
Wake-Up Call

First thing you do this morning, and every morning, is drink an 8-ounce glass of water. If you're a coffee drinker, like me, drink it black.

6:15 A.M.
Cardio

Nothing fancy on the first day. No intervals, no sprints. Just 20 to 40 minutes of straight-ahead cardio work in your preferred mode: walking, jogging, cycling, swimming, stairclimbing, whatever. Unless you're an absolute beginner, do closer to 40 minutes than 20. Set a good, fat-burning pace and keep it up. Get in some stretching when you're through.

7:00 A.M.
Ab Work

Start off with three sets of 25 Owen crunches for your upper abs, followed by three sets of 25 reverse rollups for your lower abs.

7:30 A.M.
Breakfast

A protein smoothie is a breakfast option just about every morning, starting today. Your other choice is scrambled egg whites, with one piece of toast. Drink 8 ounces of water with your breakfast.

10:00 A.M.
Mid-Morning Mini-Meal

Have a protein bar, with 12 ounces of water.

12:30 P.M.
Lunch

Eat a chicken breast with steamed green beans or asparagus, and ½ cup brown rice. Drink 12 ounces of water.

3:00 P.M.
Mid-Afternoon Mini-Meal

Down another protein bar and 12 ounces of water.

5:00/5:30 P.M.
Pre-Workout Snack

Have an apple with 12 ounces of water.

6:00 P.M.
Workout

Hit your upper-back muscles (lats and traps) fairly hard during a 30- to 40-minute strength-training session. You'll feel this in your arms as well.

Start off with three kinds of pullups, doing two sets of each to burnout (that is, until you absolutely can't do another one). The three happen to be among my favorite strength movements. They are: wide-grip pullups, close-grip pullups, and underhand pullups (chinups).

Then do wide-grip lat pulldowns, followed by close-grip lat pulldowns with your palms facing each other (a little easier with a shorter range of motion, so use more weight). Do three sets of each, 10 to 12 reps per set.

Finally, perform four sets (12 to 15 reps each) of T-bar rows, switching after each set from the palms-facing handles to the palms-down handles and back again, so that you end up doing two sets with each grip.

7:30 P.M.
Dinner

Bake or sauté some fish and serve it up with squash or zucchini, no rice. Your beverage is—you guessed it—12 ounces of water.

10:00 P.M.
Late-Night Treat

Optional: five whole unsalted, raw cashews or almonds. Not optional: 12 ounces of water.

DAY-1 EXERCISE LOG

CARDIO (A.M.)	Min	Mode	Min Completed
Steady pace	20–40		
Stretch			

AB WORK (A.M.)	Reps	Reps Completed	
Owen crunch			
Set 1	25		
Set 2	25		
Set 3	25		
Reverse rollup			
Set 1	25		
Set 2	25		
Set 3	25		

UPPER-BACK WORKOUT (P.M.)	Reps	Weight	Reps Completed
Wide-grip pullup			
Set 1	Burnout		
Set 2	Burnout		
Close-grip pullup			
Set 1	Burnout		
Set 2	Burnout		
Underhand pullup (chinup)			
Set 1	Burnout		
Set 2	Burnout		
Wide-grip lat pulldown			
Set 1	10–12		
Set 2	10–12		
Set 3	10–12		
Close-grip lat pulldown with palms facing each other			
Set 1	10–12		
Set 2	10–12		
Set 3	10–12		
T-bar row			
Set 1 (palms facing)	12–15		
Set 2 (palms down)	12–15		
Set 3 (palms facing)	12–15		
Set 4 (palms down)	12–15		

Protein Smoothie

This will be your trusted choice for many a meal to come, so let's make it right. The standard way to prepare a great protein smoothie is to run the following ingredients through your blender.

→ **½ banana.** This will go down to ¼ as time marches on. On occasion, I'll suggest frozen strawberries instead. When a smoothie shows up after noon, forgo the fruit entirely.

→ **1 cup soy milk.** Starting on Day 5 of the Tweak, you'll switch to water—or make it with water now if you're especially gung-ho.

→ **2 scoops protein powder.** It should be whey protein, easily available in a can at health food stores, drugstores, even supermarkets. Make sure it's low in carbs (about 2 grams) and sugar. The protein content will typically be about 17.5 grams per scoop.

→ **1 tablespoon natural peanut butter.** This is the kind you have to stir up to mix the peanut oil back in. If the label says it's natural, it shouldn't include sugar or added salt, but read the ingredients list to make sure.

Scrambled Egg Whites

→ Use three to five eggs if you're a big guy.

→ Separate each egg white by cracking the eggshell and then passing the yolk back and forth between the two halves while the white part falls into a bowl below.

→ You can use one of the yolks if you like.

→ Season the raw eggs with any spice you like—oregano, tarragon, whatever. But no salt. No garlic salt, either (it's mostly salt). Use a fork to whip the egg whites for a few seconds.

→ For no-stick cooking, heat 1 tablespoon flaxseed oil or olive oil in a pan over medium heat. No other kind of oil, and no butter.

→ Chop a tomato or any green vegetable, and sauté it in the pan. Chopped onions are good, too. Cook them at the same time.

→ Pour in the egg whites, then reduce the heat to low. Stir until the scrambled eggs are dry enough for your taste.

Toast

Yeah, I know, you already know how to make toast. But I have some rules for you.

→ Choose whole wheat bread. Make sure it says WHOLE WHEAT (not just WHEAT) on the label.

→ Don't spread on any butter, cream cheese, honey, jam, or anything else. Eat it dry.

→ Have one piece only. Later in the 14-day program, you'll be allowed zero pieces, so enjoy your solo slice while you can.

Protein Bar

You'll see more of these little guys in the next 2 weeks than you will your own . . . well, fill in the blank. Don't grab just any old bar off the shelf. Many products are high-carb "energy" bars—just the opposite of what you want. Check the ingredients list on the label, which looks like the fine print of an insurance contract. Here are the non-negotiable requirements.

→ It must be a *protein* bar. That means it should contain at least 20 grams of protein—preferably 30 to 40 grams.

→ Make sure it's very low in carbohydrates: no more than 4 grams, preferably 2.

→ Make extra sure it's low in sugar.

Chicken Breast

We're really talking about half of what's often sold as a chicken breast. Fowl is double-breasted, which causes confusion sometimes. You want a serving that's about the size of your hand. It may be 8 ounces, which gives you about 70 grams of protein. Just make sure the skin and bones have been removed; you can buy it packaged that way, or the butcher will do it for you.

→ To bake it, preheat the oven to 375°F.

→ Season the chicken with balsamic vinegar and/or lemon juice, as well as your favorites spices (assuming your favorite isn't salt). Onions and minced garlic are good.

→ No sauce, cream, gravy, ketchup, or soy sauce.

→ Place the chicken in a baking pan and put it on the top rack of the oven.

→ Let it cook, turning it over once, for 20 to 25 minutes, or until a thermometer inserted in the thickest portion registers 160°F and the juices run clear.

Or just heat 1 tablespoon olive oil in a skillet over medium-high heat, throw in the chicken, and let it cook for about 5 minutes on each side. If it's white all the way through, it's done. If it's pink somewhere, it's not.

Green Beans

If they're frozen, cook them according to the package directions. If they're fresh, it's best to steam them.

→ Use a pot with a lid that fits tightly. Pour in water to just below the level of the steamer (the metal thing with all the holes in it that un-folds to the circumference of the pot and holds the vegetables).

→ Bring the water to a boil over high heat.

→ Grab a handful of green beans, wash them off, season them with any spice other than salt, and lay them on the steamer.

→ Cover the pot, and let the beans steam until they're soft enough for your taste.

→ Eat 'em the way they come out—no butter, cream, sauces, et cetera.

You can also sauté the beans in a pan with fresh minced garlic and onions, cooking them over medium heat with 1 tablespoon olive or flaxseed oil.

Asparagus

Scrape off the extra-hard outer layers of the stalks if you like. Season them with spices. Lay off the butter, salt, sauces, or other condiments (in-cluding the mayonnaise you dipped those spears in when you were a kid). Then steam them just like green beans. They'll probably take longer to soften up, though.

Brown Rice

We're talking whole grain rice here, unprocessed, with all the fiber and nutrients intact. The package will tell you how to cook it. So will I.

→ Pour $2\frac{1}{3}$ cups water into a pot for every cup of dry rice. Here's a tip that will save you some hassle later on: Make enough brown rice on Day 1 to last a week—that would be $2\frac{1}{2}$ cups. Then you can reheat it as needed. At the start of the second Tweak week, Day 8, you can make 1 cup rice.

→ Put your seasoning right in the water. Use a bay leaf, pepper, turmeric—anything but salt. You can also add chopped onions, minced garlic, or even a chopped vegetable.

→ Bring the water to a boil before adding the rice.

→ Once the rice is in there, cover the pan with a tight-fitting lid, reduce the heat to a very low flame, and leave it to simmer for 45 minutes, or until all the water has been absorbed by the rice.

→ Don't add butter or oil or salt—not even if the package tells you to.

Baked or Sautéed Fish

Cooking fish is much easier than a lot of guys think. There are tons of fish to choose from: swordfish, sea bass, salmon, any white fish. Most deliver between 5 and 8 grams of protein per ounce. Buy a fillet cut so you don't have to bother with bones. Here's how I bake it.

(continued on page 200)

→ Preheat the oven to 350°F.

→ Put the fish on a piece of aluminum foil big enough that you can wrap it up like a present.

→ Season it with olive oil, lemon juice, crushed garlic, and something from your spice rack (not salt).

→ If you're having a vegetable with the fish (which you usually are), you can chop it up, season it, and put it in the tin foil to cook along with the fish.

→ Fold up the aluminum foil, making sure the oil and juice can't spill out, and cook it in the oven for 15 minutes, or until the fish flakes easily. (If the fish is salmon, cook it until it's opaque.)

If you prefer to cook your fish in a pan, it's just as easy.

→ Put the oil in the pan instead of on the fish, and heat it over medium heat.

→ Season the fish just as if you were going to bake it.

→ Throw the fish into the pan and cook it for 5 minutes or so on each side (maybe a little more or less, depending on how thick it is), again, until it flakes easily or becomes opaque.

→ You can sauté your vegetables right along with the fish. Onions are always good, but whatever vegetable you're having for this meal will work.

Squash or Zucchini

Zucchini is a type of squash, so you prepare them just the same.

→ You can steam them whole or cut up. Season them first, and don't let them steam too long. They'll get soggy. Keep in mind that as long as they're covered, vegetables keep steaming and getting softer, even after you turn off the heat.

"Never in a million years would I advise you to immediately and permanently swear off any food you like."

The Exercises

OWEN CRUNCH

1 Lie faceup on the floor with your knees up and together, your heels tucked in tight to your butt, and your feet flat on the floor and pigeon-toed. Let your fingers lightly touch the back of your head.

2 Without pulling your head with your hands, lift your shoulder blades off the floor. Then lower them back down. Keep your lower back in contact with the floor throughout.

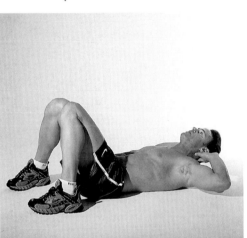

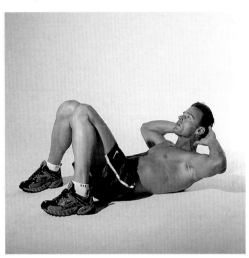

REVERSE ROLLUP

1 Lie faceup on the floor with your hands at your sides, your thighs pointing up, and your lower legs parallel to the floor.

2 Use your lower abs to roll your knees toward your chin as your butt rises off the floor. Squeeze your abs at the top, then slowly lower, one vertebra at a time.

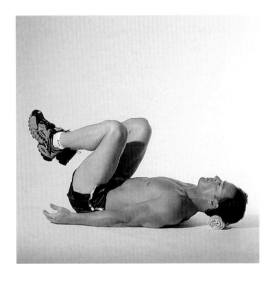

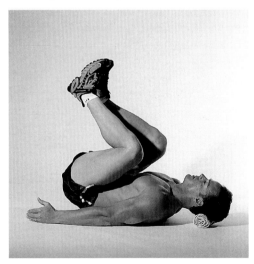

WIDE-GRIP PULLUP

1 Grab a pullup bar with an overhand grip, your hands more than shoulder-width apart. Hang so that your elbows are just ever-so-slightly bent. Bend your knees and cross your feet behind you.

2 Concentrating on your upper-back muscles, pull yourself up until your chin passes the bar. Hold this top position for a beat, then lower your body with control.

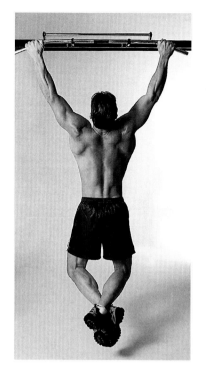
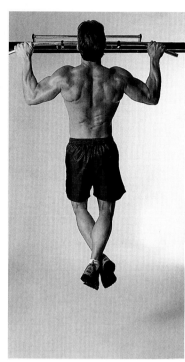

CLOSE-GRIP PULLUP

1 Grab a pullup bar with an overhand grip, your hands shoulder-width apart or less. Hang with your knees bent and your feet crossed behind you.

2 Pull yourself up until your chin passes the bar. Hold this top position for a beat, then lower your body with control.

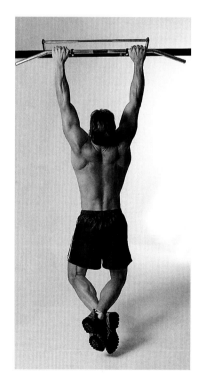
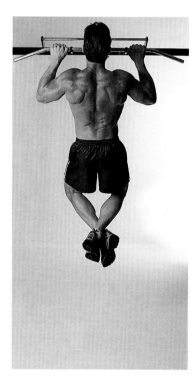

UNDERHAND PULLUP (CHINUP)

1 Grab the pullup bar with an underhand grip, your hands about shoulder-width apart or closer. Hang with your knees bent and your feet crossed behind you.

2 Pull yourself up until your chin passes the bar. Hold this top position for a beat, then lower your body with control.

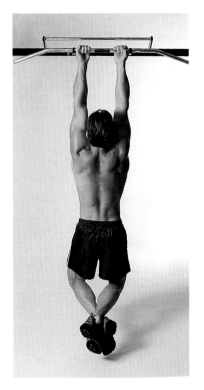 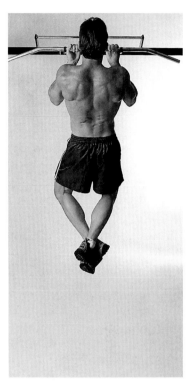

WIDE-GRIP LAT PULLDOWN

1 With an overhand grip, grab the lat-pulldown bar toward the ends so your hands are more than shoulder-width apart. Hold it with your arms straight up as you sit on the seat, facing the weight stack.

2 Pinch your shoulder blades behind you and focus on using your upper-back muscles to bring the bar to your chest, rocking your upper body back slightly from the hips. Pause, then keep working hard as you slowly let the bar back up. Proudly stick out your chest throughout.

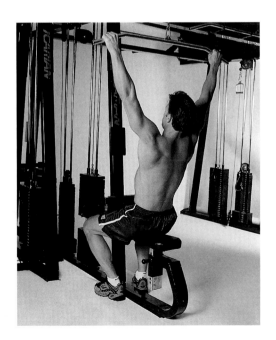 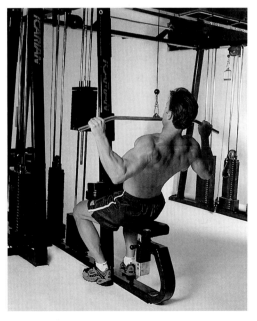

CLOSE-GRIP LAT PULLDOWN WITH PALMS FACING EACH OTHER

1 Attach the triangle handle to the lat-pulldown cable and grip it with your palms facing each other. Hold it at arm's length above you as you sit facing the weight stack.

2 Pull the handle to your chest, rocking slightly back at the end. Keep resisting as you slowly let it back up.

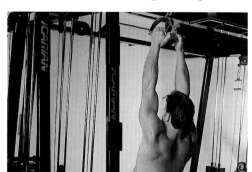
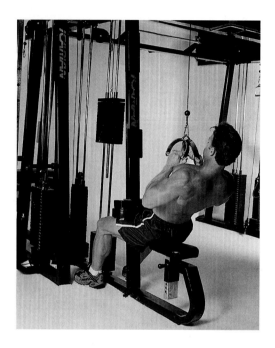

T-BAR ROW

1 Sit or stand at the T-bar station with your chest against the pad. Reach in front of you to grab the palms-facing handles.

2 Focus on your upper-back muscles as you pull the handles toward your torso, letting your elbows move behind you. Pause, then slowly return to the starting position. Complete a set, then switch to the palms-down handles.

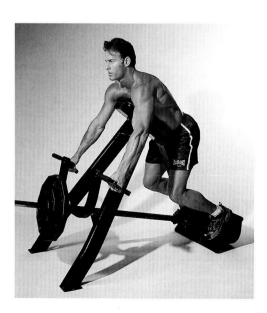
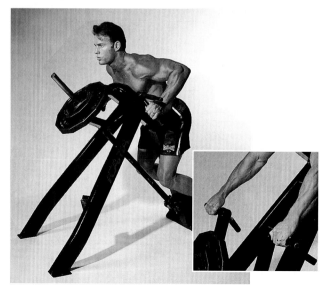

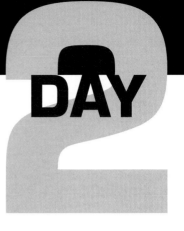

DAY 2

Now that you're off and running, let's talk about sleep. You need lots.

Remember, it's during rest that your muscle fibers grow. And if you haven't noticed already, you'll soon see that you'll have no trouble falling asleep earlier. The stepped-up workouts guarantee it.

So I'm taking the late-night snack off the schedule. If you really want one, stick to those five (no more) unsalted, raw almonds or cashews. I'm betting you'll be so tired after today's workouts that after dinner you'll pass out before you get hungry again.

The earlier you crash, the easier it will be to wake up on time. That's the way it should be. Sounder sleep is one of your weapons in this 2-week pit session.

Speaking of tiredness, don't be surprised if you feel it *before* your afternoon weight session today. Suck it up. The apple you'll eat as a pre-workout snack will deliver the energy carbs you need to hit the weights with a vengeance.

Finally, about dinner: Did it seem a tad skimpy last night? Good. Dinner shouldn't be your biggest meal of the day. Remember, it's just one of five meals (or six, if you count the pre-workout snack). Tonight, in fact, dinner will be a protein smoothie—no more, no less. Have it as early as you can, and as soon after your weight workout as possible.

6:00 A.M.
Wake-Up Call

Drink 8 ounces of water, and coffee with no sugar or cream.

6:15 A.M.
Cardio

It's the same as yesterday: 20 to 40 crisp, steady minutes in the mode of your choice.

7:00 A.M.
Ab Work

Repeat the two exercises you did yesterday: Owen crunches and reverse rollups. Take each down to two sets of 25 reps each. Then throw in alternating elbow-to-knee bicycle crunches, two sets of 40. Allow yourself very little rest between sets in this workout.

7:30 A.M.
Breakfast

Make a protein smoothie this morning if you went with the scrambled egg whites yesterday. If you had the smoothie yesterday, go for the egg whites. (See "Kitchen Tactics" on page 198.)

10:00 A.M.
Mid-Morning Mini-Meal

Have a protein bar with 12 ounces of water. If you stocked up on lots of protein bars to get you through the Tweak (not a bad idea), you may have tossed in a few that are a little higher in carbs than others. The earlier in the day you eat those higher-carb bars, the better. And if you accidentally picked up a high-carb energy bar (some have more than 50 grams of carbs), give it away to your mail carrier.

12:30 P.M.
Lunch

The featured choice today is baked or sautéed fish (see "Kitchen Tactics" on page 199) with broccoli. If you're not a big fish fan and you consider it cruel-and-unusual punishment to eat it twice in 2 days, make yourself a chicken salad. With either choice, have ½ cup of the brown rice you cooked yesterday, along with 12 ounces of water.

2:30 P.M.
Mid-Afternoon Mini-Meal

Whip up a protein smoothie (see "Kitchen Tactics" on page 198), with no banana in it. Generally speaking, leave the fruit out of any smoothie you drink in the afternoon or at night. Reason: sugar. Drink 12 ounces of water.

5:00 P.M.
Pre-Workout Snack

Bite into an apple, with 12 ounces of water. For the first few Tweak days, your pre-workout snack can be an exception to the P.M. sugar ban. Natural fruit sugar will give you a lift before you lift.

6:00 P.M.
Workout

Do a 30- to 40-minute weight-training session emphasizing your chest and legs by alternating upper- and lower-body movements. Use dumbbells rather than a barbell for the bench presses. Dumbbells keep your shoulders and elbows in more natural positions during the movements.

Start with three sets of 20 to 25 reps each of dumbbell bench presses; then switch to squats, three sets of 15 reps each.

Next do incline dumbbell bench presses (three sets of 10 to 12 reps each) to shift more

Broccoli

As with most vegetables, a typical serving of broccoli is a cup. As far as I'm concerned, you can pretty much eat as much as you want (within reason). Just save room for your protein.

Spice and steam the broccoli just like you did the green beans or asparagus on Day 1 (see "Kitchen Tactics" on page 199). Just a few minutes will do the trick. There's nothing worse than squishy broccoli.

Or if you're baking fish, put the broccoli in the tin foil and let the fish and vegetables cook together. You can also double up if you're sautéing your seafood: Simply cook the broccoli in olive oil, right along with the fish.

Chicken Salad

This is just what it sounds like: a salad with chicken in it. But it's not what they serve down at Ralph and Bessie's Country Kitchen, where an ice-cream scoop of a chickenlike substance that's mostly mayonnaise sits atop translucent lettuce. Throw away the mayo and buy yourself a tasty mix of assorted dark greens, preferably the bagged kind you don't have to wash first. Then do this:

→ Sauté a chicken breast and then cut it into strips, or bake a breast and then shred it.

→ Mix the chicken with the greens to make a generous bowlful.

→ Add some chopped raw vegetables. I like bell peppers and tomatoes. Anything green is fine. Stay away from corn and beets during the Tweak. They're high in sugar.

→ Dress your salad with a mix of balsamic vinegar, 1 tablespoon olive oil, and lots of spices. These days it's pretty easy to find natural spice blends that leave out salt and artificial ingredients. As always, shun soy sauce, creamy dressings, or anything like that. Stick with the vinegar and spices.

work to the upper part of your chest muscles (pecs). Follow with three sets of walking lunges, each set consisting of 12 to 15 reps with each leg.

Then it's back to dumbbell presses, this time on the decline bench (three sets of 12 to 15 reps each) for more emphasis on your lower pecs.

Finish up with lying hamstring curls, three sets of 12 to 15. You can substitute Romanian deadlifts for the hamstring curls, with the same sets and reps. If you have any lower-back issues, stick with the curls.

Follow up your weight work with 10 minutes of stretching.

7:00/7:30 P.M.

Dinner

No chewing tonight. Have a protein smoothie, even if you had one for breakfast. (I down two smoothies a day quite often.) Skip the banana and add a second tablespoon of peanut butter (that ups the protein count by about 4 grams). And throw in ⅓ cup of raw oat bran (reaping another 8 grams of protein and plenty of fiber). All told, there's about 55 grams of protein in this big boy.

DAY-2 EXERCISE LOG

CARDIO (A.M.)	Min	Mode	Min Completed
Steady pace	20–40		

AB WORK (A.M.)	Reps	Reps Completed	
Owen crunch			
Set 1	25		
Set 2	25		
Reverse rollup			
Set 1	25		
Set 2	25		
Alternating elbow-to-knee bicycle crunch			
Set 1	40		
Set 2	40		

"You absolutely cannot get washboard abs without consistent cardio work."

DAY-2 EXERCISE LOG

UPPER-BACK AND LEGS WORKOUT (P.M.)	Reps	Weight	Reps Completed
Dumbbell bench press			
Set 1	20–25		
Set 2	20–25		
Set 3	20–25		
Squat			
Set 1	15		
Set 2	15		
Set 3	15		
Incline dumbbell bench press			
Set 1	10–12		
Set 2	10–12		
Set 3	10–12		
Walking lunge			
Set 1	12–15 (each leg)		
Set 2	12–15 (each leg)		
Set 3	12–15 (each leg)		
Decline dumbbell bench press			
Set 1	12–15		
Set 2	12–15		
Set 3	12–15		
Lying hamstring curl (or Romanian deadlift)			
Set 1	12–15		
Set 2	12–15		
Set 3	12–15		
Stretch (10 min)			

The Exercises

OWEN CRUNCH

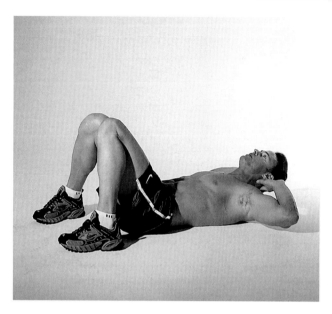
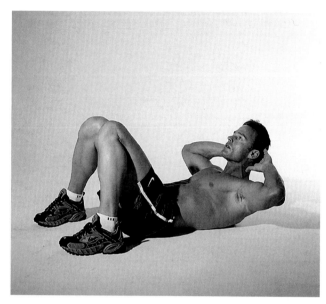

REVERSE ROLLUP

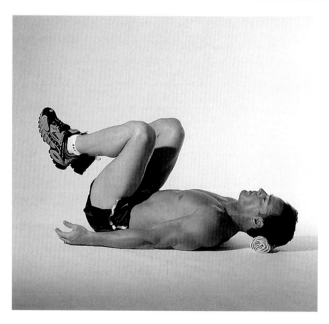
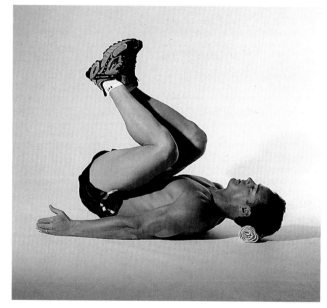

ALTERNATING ELBOW-TO-KNEE BICYCLE CRUNCH

1 Lie faceup on the floor with your back flat, your knees bent, and your fingers lightly touching the back of your head. Lifting your shoulders off the floor and twisting your torso, move your right elbow and left knee toward each other.

2 Then move your left elbow and right knee toward each other. Continue to alternate, keeping your shoulders and feet off the floor.

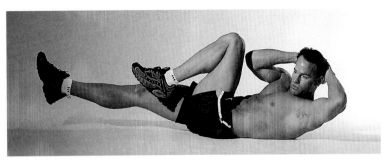

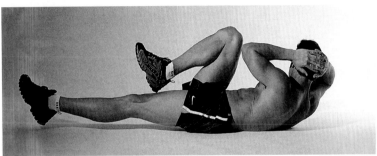

DUMBBELL BENCH PRESS

1 Lying faceup on a flat bench, hold two dumbbells up over your mid-chest with an overhand grip and straight arms.

2 Lower the weights to your armpits. Pause, then press them back up until they're almost touching above you.

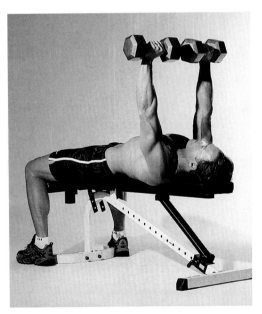

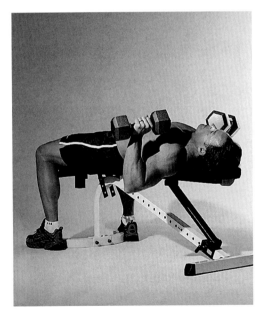

SQUAT

1 Stand with your feet no wider than shoulder-width apart and hold a loaded barbell behind you on your traps (not on the base of your neck).

2 Lower yourself from the hips until your thighs are parallel to the floor. Pause, then push yourself back to the starting position. Keep your torso straight and your knees pointing ahead throughout.

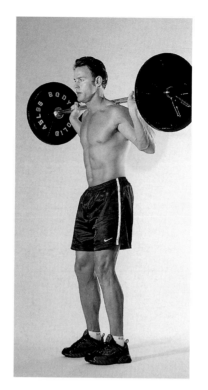
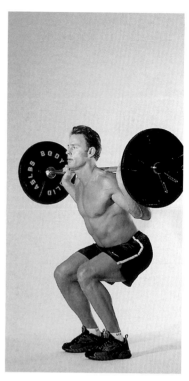

INCLINE DUMBBELL BENCH PRESS

1 Lie faceup on a bench inclined at about 45 degrees, and with arms extended, hold the dumbbells up over your collarbone or chin.

2 Perform the presses as you would on a flat bench, lowering the weights to your armpits. Pause, then push the dumbbells straight up, not out.

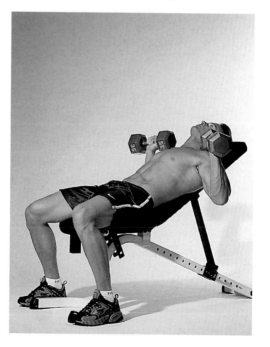

WALKING LUNGE

1 Grab a pair of dumbbells and hold them at your sides. Stand with your feet hip-width apart at one end of your house or gym.

2 Lunge forward with your nondominant leg (your left if you're right-handed), bending your knee 90 degrees. Your other knee should also bend and almost touch the floor.

Stand and bring your back foot up next to your front foot, then repeat with your dominant leg lunging forward. That's one repetition. Continue until you've completed half of your repetitions in this direction. Then turn and do the same number of walking lunges back to your starting point.

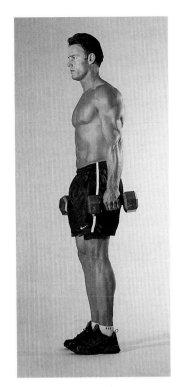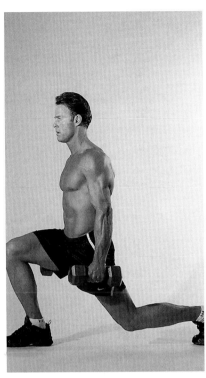

DECLINE DUMBBELL BENCH PRESS

1 Grab a pair of dumbbells and lie faceup on a decline bench with your feet under the leg supports. Hold the dumbbells just outside your shoulders, with your arms bent and your palms facing forward.

2 Push the weights straight up until your arms are extended. Lower the weights back to your chest, and pause before repeating.

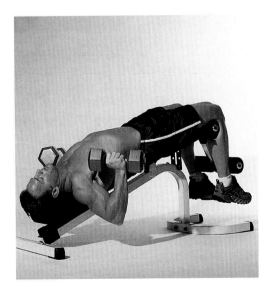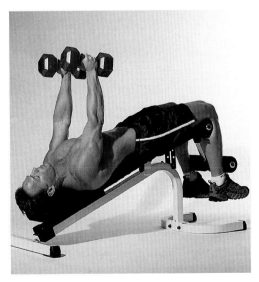

LYING HAMSTRING CURL

1 Lie facedown in a leg-curl machine with your legs extended so your Achilles tendons are hooked beneath the foot pads.

2 Bring your heels toward your butt. Pause, then slowly return to the starting position.

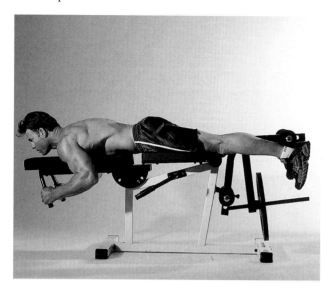
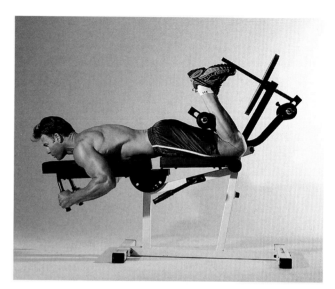

ROMANIAN DEADLIFT

1 Grab a barbell with an overhand grip that's just beyond shoulder-width. Stand holding the bar at arm's length, resting it on the fronts of your thighs. Keep your feet shoulder-width apart, your knees slightly bent, and your eyes focused straight ahead. Pull your shoulders back.

2 Slowly bend at the wasit as you lower the bar to just below your knees. Don't change the angle of your knees. Keep your head and chest up and your lower back arched. Lift your torso back to the starting position, keeping the bar as close to your body as possible.

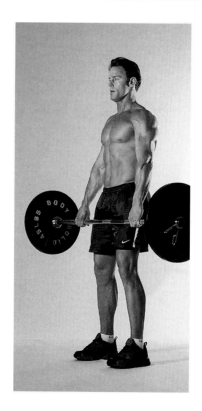
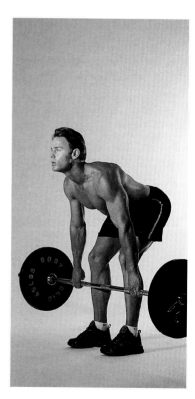

DAY 3

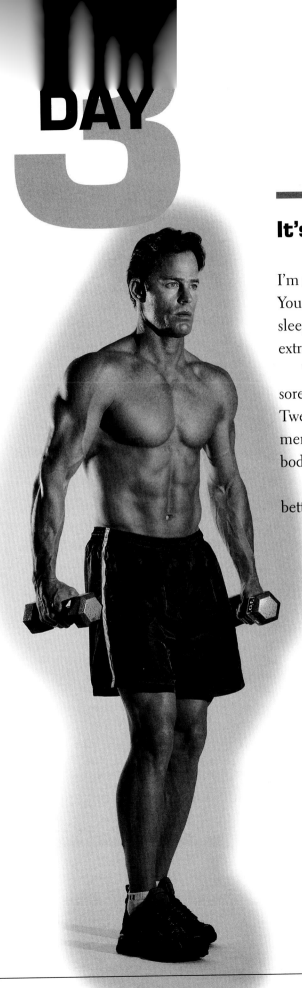

It's time to rise and whine.

I'm still setting 6:00 A.M. as your wake-up call. You may start waking up earlier as you go to sleep earlier. That's good. You no doubt need the extra time in the morning anyway.

What's probably more on your mind is how sore you feel. Day 3 is when most 2-Week Tweakers really start feeling it. No matter. Remember that pain is just weakness leaving your body. Get up in the A.M. and kick some ass.

Here's some news that may make you feel better: no ab work today!

6:00 A.M.
Wake-Up Call
Down 8 ounces of water, and coffee with no cream or sugar.

6:15 A.M.
Cardio
Do straight-ahead cardio again, for 30 to 40 minutes. (If you did just 20 minutes the first 2 days, move up to 30.) You know the drill. Believe me, I know that your legs are probably screaming at you right about now. Suck it up. It's worth it. Then stretch for 10 to 15 minutes afterward.

7:30 A.M.
Breakfast
Today it's hot oat bran. It's high in protein and fiber, and it helps your body burn fat. It will also keep you feeling full longer. Drink 12 ounces of water.

10:00 A.M.
Mid-Morning Snack
Have a protein smoothie (see "Kitchen Tactics" on page 198) or a protein bar, with 12 ounces of water.

12:30 P.M.
Lunch
Today is red-meat day. Cook 4 to 8 ounces of lean red meat, and accompany it with spinach or edamame. You can also have ½ cup brown rice. Don't forget the 12 ounces of water.

3:00 P.M.
Mid-Afternoon Mini-Meal
Again, grab a protein smoothie or a protein bar, with 12 ounces of water.

5:00/5:30 P.M.
Pre-Workout Snack
It's time for your usual apple and 12 ounces of water. If you don't feel the need for a carb-and-natural-sugar boost, but you still want a snack, go the protein-and-fat route by eating five whole unsalted cashews or almonds. Who can eat just five cashews? You can, because you want to blow everybody away on Day 14 more than you want five more nuts.

6:00 P.M.
Workout
Today's weight session calls for more sets than usual, so it may take you 45 minutes or more. It hits your shoulders and triceps. Start off with three shoulder moves:

→ Alternating dumbbell single-arm overhead press with a twist: three sets of 12 reps

→ Side lateral raise: three sets of 12 reps

→ Front deltoid raise: three sets of 12 to 15 reps

Then do three sets of standing upright rows, raising the number of reps with each set, from 12 to 15 to 20, and dropping the weight each time.

Next, to the triceps. Do three burnout sets of dips. After that, do standing triceps pushdowns (three sets of 15 reps).

Finish up with lying triceps kickbacks. Do four burnout sets, dropping the weight each time. Typically, you might go from 12 pounds to 10 to 8 to 5.

Follow up with a 10-minute stretching routine.

7:30 P.M.
Dinner
Cook up a turkey breast, with broccoli or asparagus. Sip another 12 ounces of water.

Hot Oat Bran

You'll find packaged oat bran at health food stores and, often, in the cereal aisle of a supermarket. Though the package will include cooking directions, here's what I recommend doing.

→ Put 1/3 cup oat bran and 2/3 cup water in a saucepan, stir it up, and bring it to a boil.

→ As soon as it boils, turn the heat way down and let it simmer for 2 minutes.

→ Remove it from the flame, cover it, and let it sit for 5 minutes.

→ Slice 1/2 banana into it. (Note that on Days 8 and 9 of the 2-Week Tweak, you should use only 1/4 banana in your oat bran).

→ Instead of the banana, you can sprinkle in 1/4 cup raisins.

→ Optional: Add five raw, unsalted almonds or cashews.

→ Sugar (white and brown), milk, and honey are off-limits.

Lean Red Meat

Choose a cut with 10 percent or, preferably, less fat. T-bone, filet mignon, porterhouse, and Choice-grade ground round all qualify. Pot roast, prime rib, ground chuck, and any cut that's marbled with white are out. A 4-ounce cut will give you about 35 grams of protein. Cooking it is a breeze; it's learning to eat it without salt or any kind of sauce (including steak sauce) that's tough.

→ Preheat the broiler.

→ Season the raw meat with 1 tablespoon olive oil, spices, and some balsamic vinegar.

→ Put the meat in a baking pan that can take high heat. Shove it into the oven and let it cook for just a few minutes on each side, until a thermometer inserted in the center registers 145°F for medium-rare, 160°F for medium, or 165°F for well-done.

If you're short on patience, you can just heat 1 tablespoon olive oil in a pan over high heat, and cook the meat for just a few minutes on each side. Prepare for a smoky kitchen.

Spinach

I like it fresh. You can make a salad out of uncooked leaves by adding some spices, lemon juice, and balsamic vinegar.

If you don't like raw spinach, the best way to cook it is to steam it as follows:

→ Put enough water in a pot to come up to just below the steamer. Bring it to a boil over high heat.

→ Use a whole bunch of spinach. It will shrink a ton.

→ Season it with your favorite spices. Crushed garlic and chopped onions are good to add right into the pot with the spinach. The spinach shouldn't touch the water.

→ Cover the pot and steam the spinach for only a minute or so. If you leave it in there too long, you'll get a soggy mess. But if you steam it just a tad, you'll have a delicious, nutrient-rich side dish.

Edamame

These are the soybeans you get at Japanese restaurants. Health food stores with decent produce sections also have them. You may even find them at regular stores because they're getting popular. They come in pods, just like peas. In fact, they look like peas.

Steam a handful or two of the pods just as you would green beans (see "Kitchen Tactics" on page 199). Then just pile them on a plate, pop them open, and eat them like popcorn. Or you can shell them all after steaming and eat them with a spoon.

Most people like to squeeze lemon on their edamame. But they're great plain.

Turkey Breast

Six ounces of white meat from a turkey breast provides more than 50 grams of protein. You can buy turkey breast precooked: Just cut off a piece the size you want and heat it up in a pan or microwave oven. If you buy raw turkey breast from your butcher, prepare it the same way you would a chicken breast (see "Kitchen Tactics" on page 198). Make sure the skin is off.

DAY-3 EXERCISE LOG

CARDIO (A.M.)	Min	Mode	Min Completed
Steady pace	30–40		

Stretch (10–15 min)

SHOULDERS AND TRICEPS WORKOUT (P.M.)	Reps	Weight	Reps Completed
Alternating dumbbell single-arm overhead press with a twist			
Set 1	12		
Set 2	12		
Set 3	12		
Side lateral raise			
Set 1	12		
Set 2	12		
Set 3	12		
Front deltoid raise			
Set 1	12–15		
Set 2	12–15		
Set 3	12–15		
Standing upright row			
Set 1	12		
Set 2 (drop)	15		
Set 3 (drop)	20		
Dip			
Set 1	Burnout		
Set 2	Burnout		
Set 3	Burnout		
Standing triceps pushdown			
Set 1	15		
Set 2	15		
Set 3	15		
Lying triceps kickback			
Set 1	Burnout		
Set 2 (drop)	Burnout		
Set 3 (drop)	Burnout		
Set 4 (drop)	Burnout		

Stretch (10 min)

The Exercises

ALTERNATING DUMBBELL SINGLE-ARM OVERHEAD PRESS WITH A TWIST

1 Sit holding two dumbbells at your shoulders with your palms facing toward you.

2 Lift one of the weights straight up to the ceiling, rotating your wrist so your palm faces away from you at the top of the movement. Rotate back in the other direction while lowering back down. Then perform the same movement with the other arm. That's 1 rep.

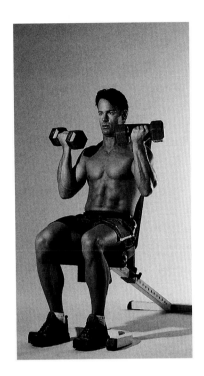 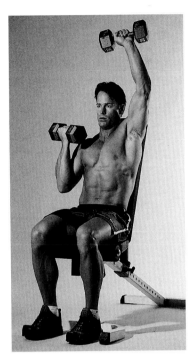

SIDE LATERAL RAISE

1 Stand or sit with a slight tilt forward from the waist. Hold two dumbbells down at your sides with your palms facing your thighs.

2 Use your shoulders to raise your arms up and out to the sides until they're parallel to the floor. Then lower to the starting position.

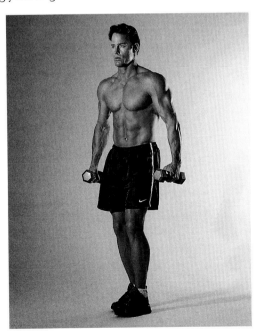 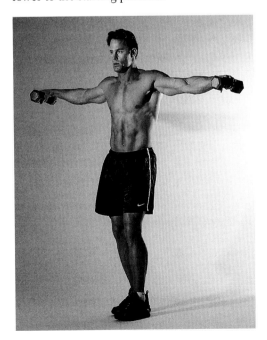

FRONT DELTOID RAISE

1 Hold two dumbbells down in front of you, palms facing forward.

2 With straight arms, raise the weights out in front of you until your upper arms are parallel to the floor. Then lower to the starting position.

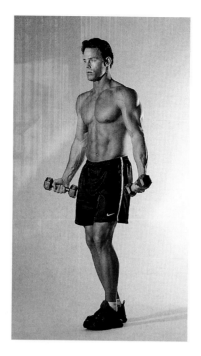
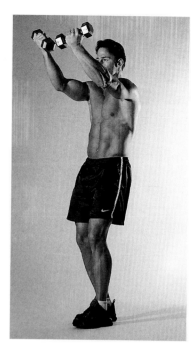

STANDING UPRIGHT ROW

1 Grab a barbell with a close, overhand grip and let it hang at arm's length in front of you as you stand up straight.

2 Pull the bar up until it's in front of your chest. Then lower to the starting position.

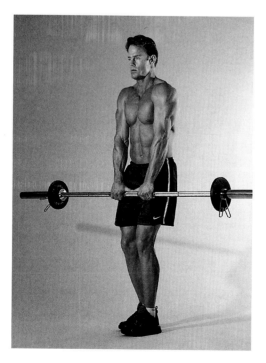
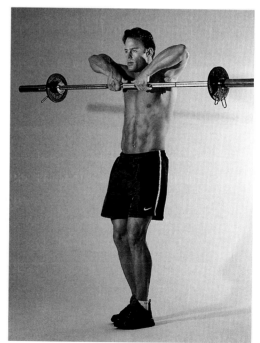

DIP

1 Grab the handles near the ends of the dip-station bars. Jump up and support your body weight with your arms. Bend your knees and cross your feet behind you.

2 Lower yourself until your upper arms are parallel to the floor. Then push yourself back up to the starting position.

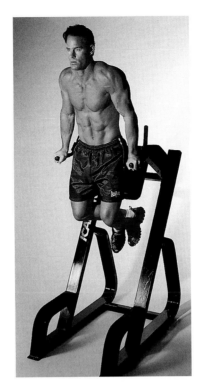 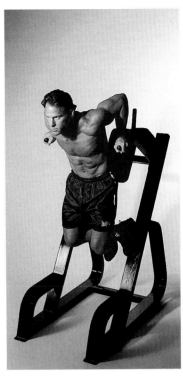

STANDING TRICEPS PUSHDOWN

1 Attach the short, straight bar to the high pulley of a cable station and grab it with an overhand grip. Stand with one foot slightly in front of the other, your elbows close to your sides, and your forearms just above parallel to the floor.

2 Without moving your upper arms, extend your forearms down until they're almost straight. Pause, then slowly return to the starting position.

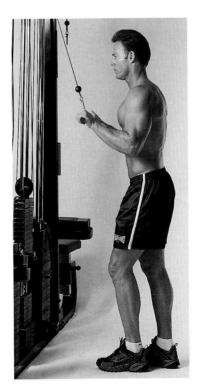 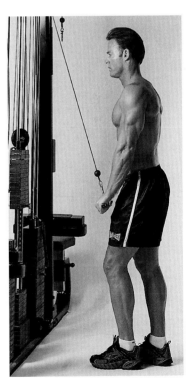

LYING TRICEPS KICKBACK

1 Lie facedown on a bench with your chin at the very edge. Bend your knees so your feet point up. Cross your feet. Keep your elbows at your sides as you let your forearms hang straight down, a light dumbbell in each hand.

2 Squeeze your shoulder blades together as your move your forearms back and up until your arms are straight. Pause, then slowly return to the starting position.

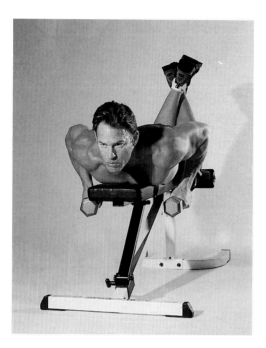 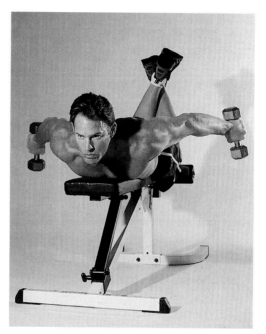

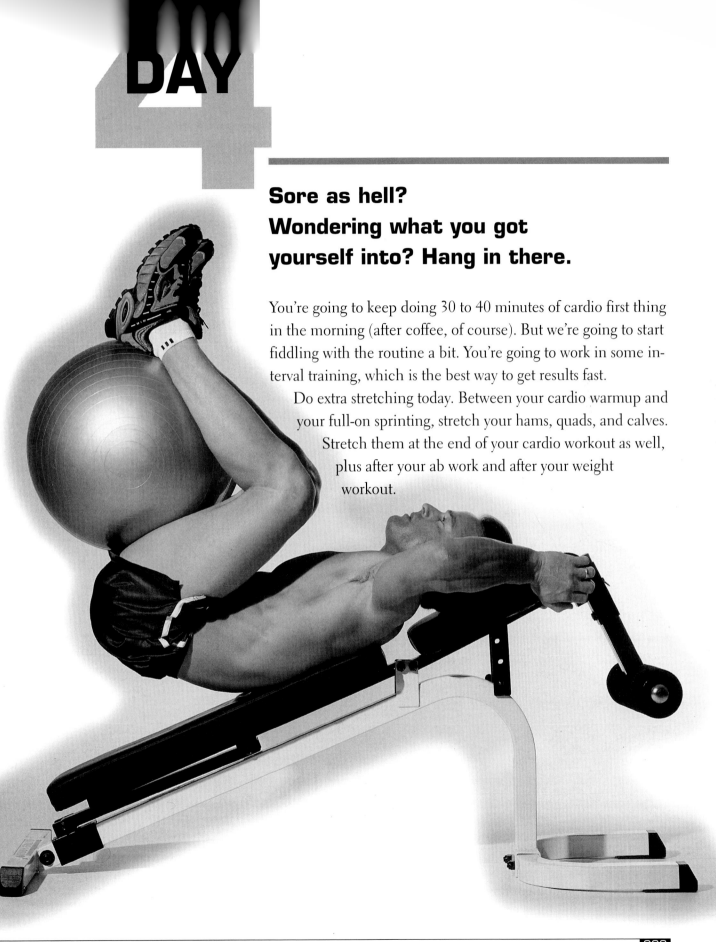

DAY 4

Sore as hell?
Wondering what you got
yourself into? Hang in there.

You're going to keep doing 30 to 40 minutes of cardio first thing in the morning (after coffee, of course). But we're going to start fiddling with the routine a bit. You're going to work in some interval training, which is the best way to get results fast.

Do extra stretching today. Between your cardio warmup and your full-on sprinting, stretch your hams, quads, and calves. Stretch them at the end of your cardio workout as well, plus after your ab work and after your weight workout.

6:00 A.M.
Wake-Up Call
Pour the usual coffee, no sugar or cream. Drink 8 ounces of water.

6:15 A.M.
Cardio
For the first half of your 30 to 40 minutes today, do whatever you've been doing for past 3 days: Walk, jog, cycle, swim laps. . . . Then do that hams, quads, and calves stretching.

For the second 15 to 20 minutes, do some interval training, which essentially means vary your pace. Run hard (slower than a sprint but faster than a jog) for 1 or 2 minutes (depending on your level of conditioning), then walk for a minute. Keep that up until your time is finished. If you don't want to get off the bike or out of the water, do the equivalent in your own mode of exercise.

If your legs are still screaming in pain from that killer leg workout 2 days ago, I'll let you keep walking or jogging for the duration, without the intervals just yet. But don't do it on a level surface. Crank up the incline on your treadmill or find a hill in your neighborhood, and attack it for at least half of your cardio time.

There's a third choice, for maniacs only. If you're really feeling cocky and you think my program so far is cake, lace up your shoes and get ready to fly. Warm up with a 10-minute jog or 10 minutes of alternating high knees (heel to butt, to the sides, and back behind you). Then crank up the treadmill incline or find a steep, long hill and sprint at about 75 percent of full effort for 30 to 40 seconds. Walk back down and do it again. Blow out as many of these sprints as you can.

Whichever option you go with, don't forget to stretch out your hams, quads, and calves afterward.

7:00 A.M.
Ab Work
Today, do three sets of 20 to 25 reverse rollups on a decline bench with a Swiss ball. Then do side jackknifes, one set to burnout on each side. Finish with two burnout sets of Owen crunches, weighted this time.

Afterward, cool down by stretching those hams, quads, and calves.

7:30 A.M.
Breakfast
You get three choices today: hot oat bran, scrambled egg whites, or a protein smoothie. You've had all of those already, so you probably know which you prefer. (I'm a smoothie man myself.) You should also have the preparation down. If not, just check back to the instructions in the "Kitchen Tactics" for the first 3 days (see page 217 for oat bran, or page 198 for the eggs or smoothie). Whichever breakfast you choose, drink at least 12 ounces of water.

10:00 A.M.
Mid-Morning Mini-Meal
Have a protein bar with 12 ounces of water.

12:30 P.M.
Lunch
It's white-meat day today. Your choices are chicken (or turkey) salad (see "Kitchen Tactics" on page 207) with ½ cup brown rice, or chicken fajitas with black beans. Also, slurp 12 ounces of water.

3:00 P.M.
Mid-Afternoon Mini-Meal
Help yourself to another protein bar or a protein smoothie, with 12 ounces of water. Keep

in mind that a smoothie will deliver more grams of protein than a bar will, along with more calories.

5:00 P.M.

Pre-Workout Snack

If you don't feel like eating another apple, have a cup of raw or lightly steamed broccoli (see "Kitchen Tactics" on page 207). Or go for the protein/fat alternative from yesterday: five un-salted, raw almonds or cashews.

6:00 P.M.

Workout

This is at least a 45-minute session that targets your upper back in much the same way you did on Day 1. You're also going to include some curls for your biceps. There's a lot to do, so let's get to it.

The first three exercises are exactly the same as on Day 1—that is, two burnout sets each of wide-grip pullups, close-grip pullups, and underhand pullups (chinups). That doesn't sound like much, but as you probably remember from Day 1, burnout sets are hell on earth. And you love it.

The next two exercises are also the same as on Day 1—three sets each of wide-grip and close-grip lat pulldowns—but up the rep count to 12 to 15 per set.

Same deal for the T-bar rows: Do four sets, alternating grips, as on Day 1; but increase your reps to 15 to 20.

Next come the curls. Lots of reps get the job done here. Do three sets of seated dumbbell curls at 21 reps apiece, dividing those 21 reps into three segments of 7 reps each. For the first 7 reps, bring the dumbbells only halfway up from the down position, then return them. For the next 7, start at the halfway position and bring them to the top. For the final 7, perform the whole range of motion, bottom to top.

After you've done that three times, finish up with two more sets of seated dumbbell curls, this time alternating arms with a twist at the top and doing 20 reps per set.

Enjoy! And round out the day's exercise with some final stretches for hams, quads, and calves.

7:30 P.M.

Dinner

Use up some more of the lettuce you bought for your chicken salad by making a tuna salad. Drink 12 ounces of water.

> *"I want you to drink water all day long—before, during, and after meals, and especially during and after your workouts."*

Chicken Fajitas

Nothing fancy here—it's just a nifty alternative to the regular baked or sautéed chicken breast.

→ Heat 1 tablespoon olive oil in a skillet over medium-high heat.

→ Add the chicken (4 to 8 ounces, depending on your size), and cook it quickly on both sides.

→ Once the chicken has cooked a bit, it's easier to cut into strips. Slice it up.

→ Add chopped green bell pepper, onions, and green chiles (optional). You can also add some chopped tomato at the last minute. Cook until the chicken is no longer pink and the juices run clear.

→ Spice it up good with anything but salt. Cumin works great.

→ No salsa, no sour cream.

→ No tortillas or tortilla chips.

Black Beans

If you get them in a can, make sure that they're not refried and that there's no added lard or salt. Your best bet is to buy dried black beans (they're pretty cheap) and cook them up yourself. Here's how.

→ If you can remember, let the beans soak for a few hours (or overnight) first. This will cut down the cooking time.

→ Drain the beans and put them in a pot with plenty of water (enough that it's three times as high as the beans).

→ You can really go to town with the flavoring. Thrown in chopped onions, crushed garlic, a bay leaf, and whatever else you like. No salt.

→ Bring the water to a boil over high heat, then reduce the heat to low, cover the pot, and let the beans simmer for a few hours, until they're soft.

If you have a pressure cooker somewhere around the kitchen, it will cook the beans in much less time. Follow the instructions in the manual that came with it (the one you threw in a drawer someplace and haven't seen since).

Tuna Salad

Like the chicken salad, this isn't a mayonnaise-and-celery concoction (although you can use celery if you like). It's a salad with tuna in it. Buy white albacore tuna; it's more expensive but much better than other kinds. Make sure it's packed in water, not oil. When you get it home from the store, do this:

→ Get the tuna out of the can and rinse it to get rid of the excess sodium.

→ Drain the tuna, then just toss it into a crisp salad of spinach or dark green lettuce, bell peppers, and perhaps some raw broccoli or steamed and cooled edamame (see "Kitchen Tactics" on page 217).

→ Dress the salad with balsamic vinegar, a little olive oil, pepper, and spices. No salt, no creamy dressings.

DAY-4 EXERCISE LOG

CARDIO (A.M.)	Min	Mode	Min Completed
OPTION 1			
Steady pace	15–20		
Stretch			
Hams			
Quads			
Calves			
Intervals	15–20		
OPTION 2			
Steady pace	15–20		
Stretch			
Hams			
Quads			
Calves			
Steady pace, incline	15–20		
OPTION 3			
Jog or high knees	10		
Stretch			
Hams			
Quads			
Calves			
30- to 40-second sprints, incline	Burnout		
STRETCH			
Hams			
Quads			
Calves			

DAY-4 EXERCISE LOG

AB WORK (A.M.)	Reps	Weight	Reps Completed
Decline reverse rollup with Swiss ball			
Set 1	20–25	N/A	
Set 2	20–25	N/A	
Set 3	20–25	N/A	
Side jackknife	Burnout (each side)	N/A	
Weighted Owen crunch			
Set 1	Burnout		
Set 2	Burnout		
Stretch			
Hams			
Quads			
Calves			

UPPER-BACK AND BICEPS WORKOUT (P.M.)	Reps	Weight	Reps Completed
Wide-grip pullup			
Set 1	Burnout		
Set 2	Burnout		
Close-grip pullup			
Set 1	Burnout		
Set 2	Burnout		
Underhand pullup (chinup)			
Set 1	Burnout		
Set 2	Burnout		
Wide-grip lat pulldown			
Set 1	12–15		
Set 2	12–15		
Set 3	12–15		
Close-grip lat pulldown with palms facing each other			
Set 1	12–15		
Set 2	12–15		
Set 3	12–15		
T-bar row			
Set 1 (palms facing)	15–20		
Set 2 (palms down)	15–20		
Set 3 (palms facing)	15–20		
Set 4 (palms down)	15–20		

DAY-4 EXERCISE LOG

UPPER-BACK AND BICEPS WORKOUT (P.M.)	Reps	Weight	Reps Completed
Seated dumbbell curl			
Set 1			
Bottom to middle	7		
Middle to top	7		
Full range	7		
Set 2			
Bottom to middle	7		
Middle to top	7		
Full range	7		
Set 3			
Bottom to middle	7		
Middle to top	7		
Full range	7		
Alternating seated dumbbell curl with a twist			
Set 1 (each arm)	20		
Set 2 (each arm)	20		
Stretch			
Hams			
Quads			
Calves			

"I do stretches all day long, just about wherever I am."

The Exercises

DECLINE REVERSE ROLLUP WITH SWISS BALL

1 Lie head-highest on a decline bench, holding on to the top of the bench or the foot pads behind you. Grip a Swiss ball between your heels and your butt.

2 Squeeze the ball as you bring your knees toward your chin as in a standard reverse rollup.

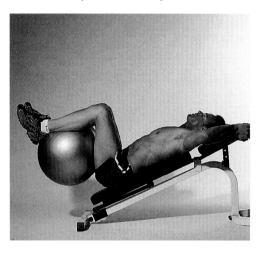
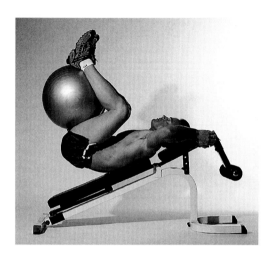

SIDE JACKKNIFE

1 Lie on your left hip, with your legs nearly straight and slightly raised off the floor. Also raise your torso off the floor, with your left forearm on the floor for balance. Hold your other hand behind your right ear, with your elbow pointed toward your feet.

2 Lift your legs toward your torso, while keeping your torso stationary. Pause to feel the contraction on the right side of your waist. Then slowly lower your legs and repeat. Finish the set on that side, then lie on your right hip and do the same number of repetitions.

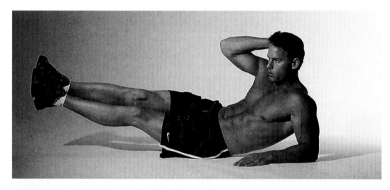
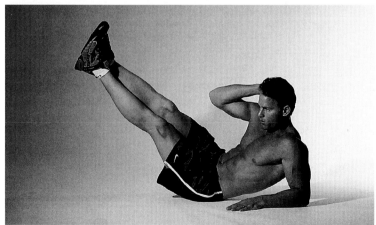

WEIGHTED OWEN CRUNCH

1 In the normal Owen-crunch starting position, hold a 5- or 10-pound weight behind your head or on your chest.

2 Perform the crunch as usual.

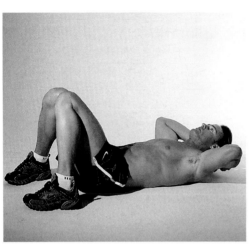

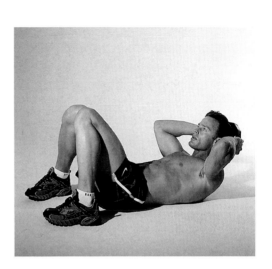

WIDE-GRIP PULLUP

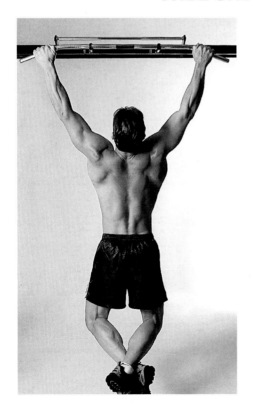

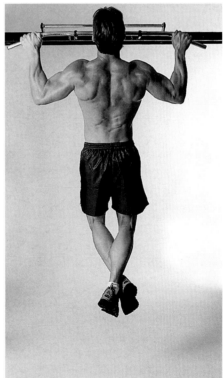

CLOSE-GRIP PULLUP

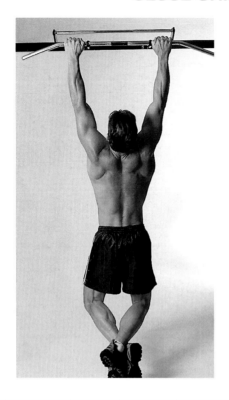 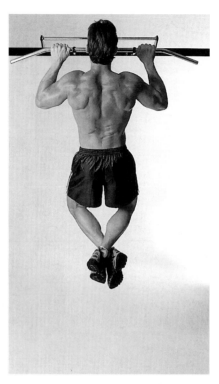

UNDERHAND PULLUP (CHINUP)

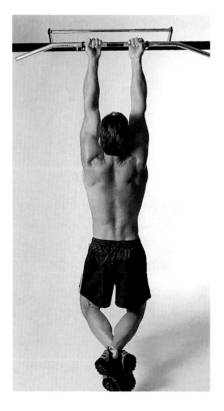 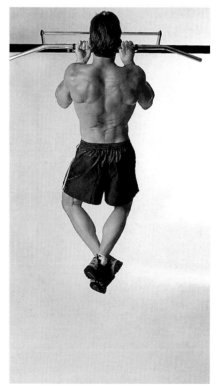

WIDE-GRIP LAT PULLDOWN

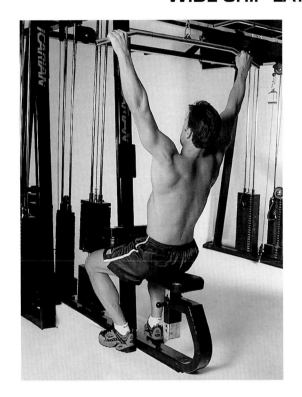 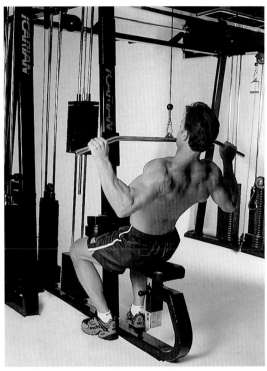

CLOSE-GRIP LAT PULLDOWN WITH PALMS FACING EACH OTHER

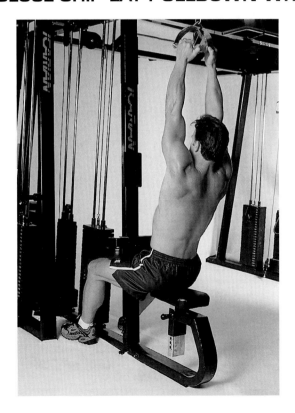 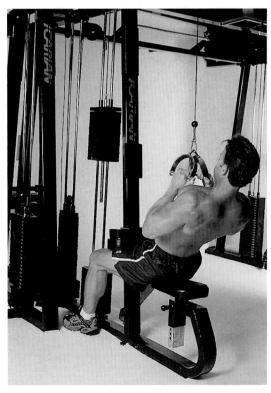

T-BAR ROW

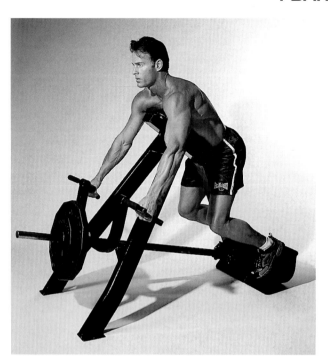

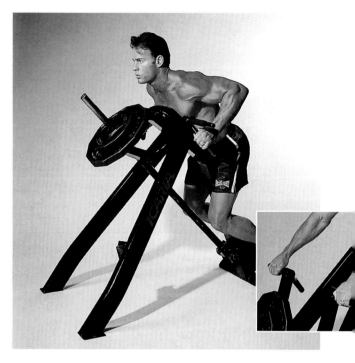

SEATED DUMBBELL CURL

1 Grab two dumbbells with an underhand grip and sit at the end of the bench, letting your arms hang straight down outside either thigh, palms facing forward.

2 Moving only your forearms, lift the weights up to your shoulders. Pause, then slowly lower to the starting position.

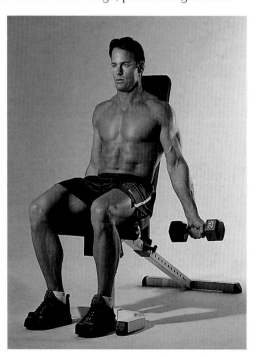

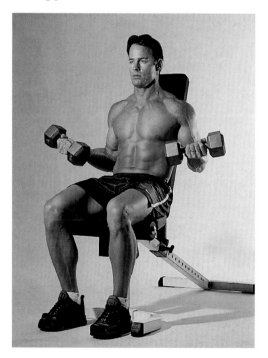

ALTERNATING SEATED DUMBBELL CURL WITH A TWIST

1 Sit holding two dumbbells down at arm's length, with your palms turned toward each other.

2 Curl just one of the weights toward your shoulder, rotating your wrist by bringing your pinkie to the outside so you finish with your palm facing you. Rotate your wrist back as you lower the weight. Then do the same thing with the other arm.

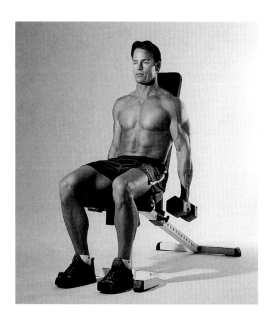

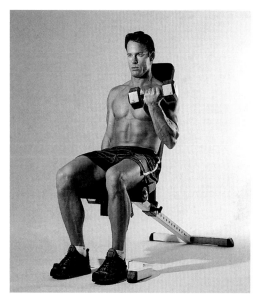

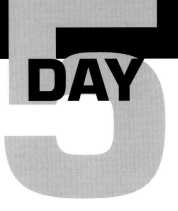

DAY 5

Go the extra mile.

Because you've been working so hard, you owe it to yourself to squeeze out every bit of additional benefit you can during these 2 weeks. If you're not already in the habit of doing so, walk as much as you can as you go about your day today (and every day).

Don't take elevators or escalators; take the stairs instead. If you have a meeting with a coworker, see if he'll agree to talk while the two of you walk outside. When parking, take whichever space in the lot is farthest away from your final destination. These little extras add up, believe it or not—even over these last 10 days of your Tweak. Taking the extra steps is a great, uplifting habit that will serve you well beyond Day 14.

By the way, though you'll start walking more, you won't do any ab work today.

6:00 A.M.
Wake-Up Call

Chug your requisite coffee without sugar or cream, plus 8 ounces of water.

6:15 A.M.
Cardio

How was that interval or sprinting routine I had you do yesterday? Challenging and invigorating? Great. Do it again today (refer back to page 224, if necessary).

Do you want another option? Try this: Walk or jog for 30 to 40 minutes, as usual, without intervals or sprints. However, every 8 to 10 minutes, stop and do a set of 20 to 25 weightless squats (see page 212; ignore the reference to the barbell) followed immediately (don't rest) by a set of walking lunges (see page 213), 15 to 20 reps per leg. Then continue your walking, jogging, or whatever until the next squat/lunge break 8 to 10 minutes later. You should be able to complete four sets of squats/lunges during your cardio session today if you choose this option.

After your cardio workout, stretch your hams, quads, calves, glutes, and groin.

7:30 A.M.
Breakfast

You get three options this morning: hot oat bran, as on Day 3 (see "Kitchen Tactics" on page 217); scrambled egg whites with vegetables; or a protein smoothie (see "Kitchen Tactics" on page 198 if you need a recipe reminder). From now on, make your smoothies with water (not soy milk). And for a change of pace, try adding 4 frozen strawberries instead of ½ banana.

As always, drink 12 ounces of water (in addition to the H_2O in the smoothie).

10:00 A.M.
Mid-Morning Mini-Meal

Keep this to a protein bar and 12 ounces of water. Remember that the bar should contain at least 20 grams of protein and very little sugar and carbs (4 grams, tops).

12:30 P.M.
Lunch

Your entrée today is the baked or sautéed chicken breast you first learned to make in "Kitchen Tactics" on page 198. For your side dish, instead of rice, have one of the following: steamed green beans or asparagus (from "Kitchen Tactics" on page 199), steamed broccoli (first introduced in "Kitchen Tactics" on page 207), or spinach steamed or in a salad (a holdover from "Kitchen Tactics" on page 217—unless you want the fancier salad at right).

Today you can go for 12 ounces of unsweetened iced tea instead of the usual water.

3:00 P.M.
Mid-Afternoon Mini-Meal

Mix up a protein smoothie, but don't put any fruit in it. Or munch a protein meal-replacement bar (a more hard-core version of your usual protein bar).

5:30 P.M.
Pre-Workout Snack

Same as yesterday: Bite into an apple or 1 cup of raw or steamed broccoli. Your no-carb pre-workout snack can now be a small, plain chicken breast. And don't forget your 12 ounces of water.

Workout

Today's routine focuses on your chest. It's not a long workout, but it's intense. Here's what to do.

Start with two sets of decline pushups to burnout. Then, before moving on, stretch your pecs.

Post–pec stretch, do three dumbbell-bench-press exercises. Start with incline and then decline presses: three sets of 10 to 12 reps for each.

Finish with plain old dumbbell bench presses, two sets of 20 reps.

Dinner

Your protein tonight is lean red meat, broiled or sautéed, just like Day 3's lunch (see "Kitchen Tactics" on page 217). With it, have another of the greens from today's lunch menu. Wash it all down with 12 ounces of water.

KITCHEN TACTICS

Fresh Spinach Salad

→ Rinse and drain an entire bunch of spinach.

→ Add ¼ cup cooked kidney beans. If they're from a can, rinse and drain them first to get rid of the extra sodium.

→ Add ¼ cup garbanzo beans, also rinsed and drained if they're from a can.

→ Add chopped tomatoes, onions, and bell peppers.

→ Top with a dressing of 1 tablespoon olive oil, some balsamic vinegar, lemon juice, and spices (no salt).

"Don't use a creamy salad dressing— that converts a healthy dish into an unhealthy one."

DAY-5 EXERCISE LOG

CARDIO (A.M.)	Min or Reps	Mode	Min or Reps Completed
OPTION 1			
Steady pace	15–20 min		
Stretch			
Hams			
Quads			
Calves			
Intervals	15–20 min		
OPTION 2			
Jog or high knees	10 min		
Stretch			
Hams			
Quads			
Calves			
30- to 40-second sprints, incline	Burnout		
OPTION 3			
Steady pace	8–10 min		
Weightless squat	20–25 reps	N/A	
Walking lunge	15–20 reps (each leg)	N/A	
Steady pace	8–10 min		
Weightless squat	20–25 reps	N/A	
Walking lunge	15–20 reps (each leg)	N/A	
Steady pace	8–10 min		
Weightless squat	20–25 reps	N/A	
Walking lunge	15–20 reps (each leg)	N/A	
Steady pace	8–10 min		
Weightless squat	20–25 reps	N/A	
Walking lunge	15–20 reps (each leg)	N/A	
STRETCH			
Hams			
Quads			
Calves			
Glutes			
Groin			

DAY-5 EXERCISE LOG

CHEST WORKOUT (P.M.)	Reps	Weight	Reps Completed
Decline pushup			
Set 1	Burnout		
Set 2	Burnout		
Pec stretch			
Incline dumbbell bench press			
Set 1	10–12		
Set 2	10–12		
Set 3	10–12		
Decline dumbbell bench press			
Set 1	10–12		
Set 2	10–12		
Set 3	10–12		
Dumbbell bench press			
Set 1	20		
Set 2	20		

"I developed my eating
and workout routine through
trial and error, keeping what
worked for my body and
discarding what didn't.
I want you to do that, too."

The Exercises

DECLINE PUSHUP

1 Put your feet up on a bench, keeping your legs straight as you support your upper body with your palms on the floor, arms straight.

2 Lower your chest almost to the floor. Then push yourself back up to the starting position.

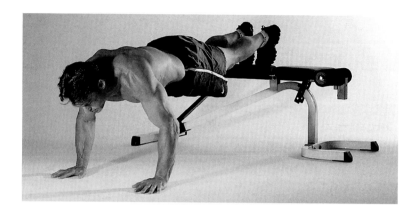

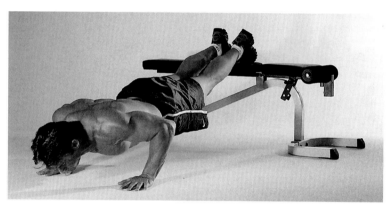

INCLINE DUMBBELL BENCH PRESS

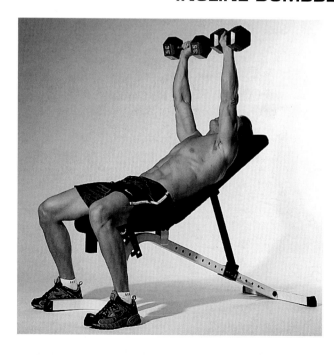

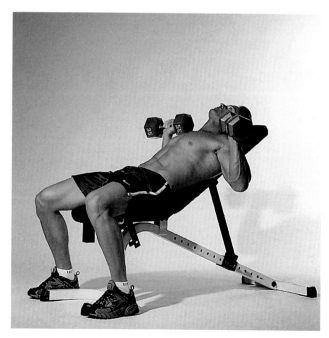

DECLINE DUMBBELL BENCH PRESS

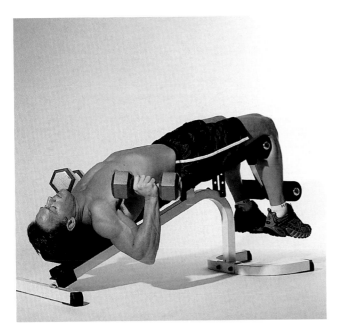
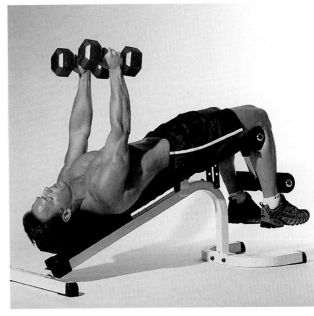

DUMBBELL BENCH PRESS

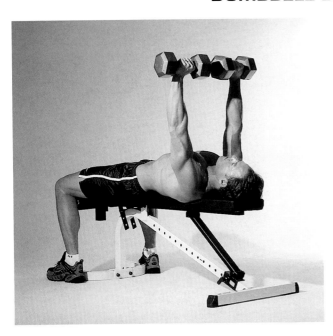
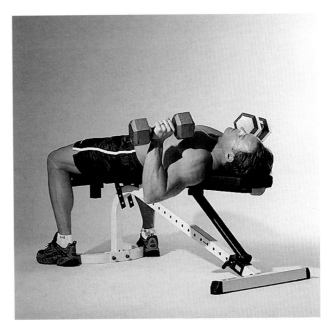

DAY

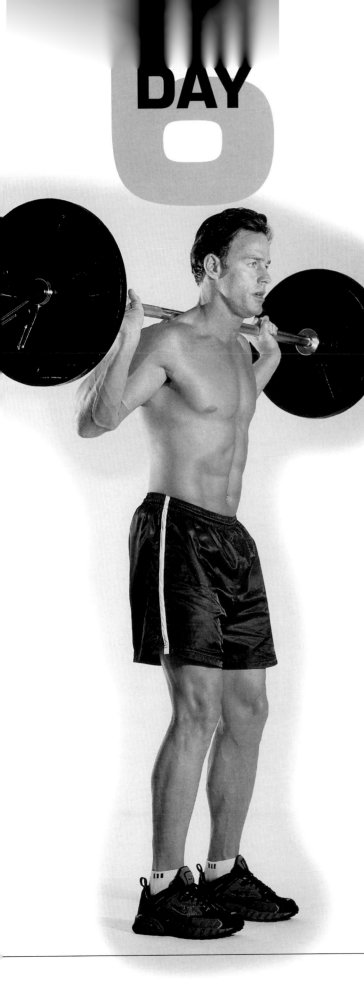

You're getting a leg up.

Your muscles may still be in a state of shock, and your legs may feel like concrete slabs sewn together with transatlantic cable. But good things are happening. Your VO_2 max is rapidly increasing from your steady cardio work, meaning you're better able to use oxygen for endurance exercise. And your increasing muscle mass is jacking up your metabolism and turning you into a fat-burning inferno.

In my book, pounding your legs is the key to fat loss. They include your biggest muscle groups, and when you use them like we're using them, they're your fat-burning engines. Long after your leg and back workouts are completed, your body continues raising your testosterone levels and burning tons of calories all day and night.

That's why I've had you working your legs so much already, even on days that focus on your upper body. So don't slack off on your legs, not even if it seems like we're overdoing it. Trust me, there's a method to my madness.

All today's meal options are compiled from the previous 5 days of the Tweak, so you won't learn any new "Kitchen Tactics."

6:00 A.M.
Wake-Up Call

You guessed it: black coffee and 8 ounces of water.

6:15 A.M.
Cardio

If you've been doing the interval or sprint workout and you love it, stick with it.

Still, it's okay if you want to mellow out today. A straight-ahead 30- to 40-minute bike ride, walk, or jog will burn those calories and spare your aching legs a bit.

7:00 A.M.
Ab Work

Perform three sets to burnout today: one set each of two familiar movements, and one new reverse-rollup variation (not in that order, however).

→ Decline reverse rollup with Swiss ball

→ Decline reverse rollup with overhead jackknife

→ Weighted Owen crunch

7:30/8:00 A.M.
Breakfast

Your choices are the same as yesterday—that is, hot oat bran (see "Kitchen Tactics" on page 217); scrambled egg whites with vegetables, or a water-based protein smoothie with either strawberries or banana (see "Kitchen Tactics" on page 198). As usual, drink 12 ounces of water.

10:00 A.M.
Mid-Morning Mini-Meal

Another protein bar. You've surely noticed by now that a high-protein (over 20 grams), low-carb (under 4 grams) bar isn't exactly a taste

treat. No matter. You're not eating a candy bar. You're feeding your muscles.

12:30 P.M.
Lunch

You're on your own today. Choose any one of the lunch suggestions from the first 5 days. (Flip back to pages 196, 206, 216, 224, and 238 to mull over those options.)

3:00 P.M.
Mid-Afternoon Mini-Meal

Rev up your blender for a good ol' protein smoothie. As always in the afternoon, don't include any fruit. And stick with the water, not soy milk. Put in the usual 1 tablespoon natural peanut butter.

5:30 P.M.
Pre-Workout Snack

If you're feeling draggy from all I've put you through this week, go for a carb boost with an apple. Otherwise, make it a protein snack, treating yourself to a small, plain baked or sautéed chicken breast (as on page 198, in "Kitchen Tactics"). Your goal is to gradually eliminate carbs—especially sugar—and since you're just about at the halfway mark, now is as good a time as any to start making some cuts.

6:00 P.M.
Workout

Today is a shoulder day, combined this time with leg work. Plan on spending about 45 minutes in the weight room today.

Start off with three supersets of these two exercises:

→ Dumbbell single-arm overhead press with a twist: 8 to 10 reps each arm (don't alternate arms this time)

→ Squat: 15–20 reps

Do 8 to 10 overhead presses with one arm, followed immediately by 8 to 10 with the other arm. Then, without rest, do the 15 to 20 squats. That's one superset. Do that three times.

The rest of your workout consists of regular sets, alternating between shoulder and leg exercises, as so:

→ T-bar row: three sets of 12 reps each

→ Walking lunge: three sets of 15 reps per leg

→ Bent-over (or seated) dumbbell rear delt raise: three sets of 15 reps

You have a choice with the last lower-body exercise: It can be either lying hamstring curls or Romanian deadlifts. For either one, do three sets of 12 to 15 reps.

7:30 P.M.

Dinner

Your best choice tonight is another protein smoothie, just the way you had it at lunch. But I won't insist on that. If you prefer, go for any of the dinner choices of the past 5 days (on pages 196, 207, 216, 225, and 239).

DAY-6 EXERCISE LOG

CARDIO (A.M.)	Min	Mode	Min Completed
OPTION 1			
Steady pace	15–20		
Stretch			
Hams			
Quads			
Calves			
Intervals	15–20		
OPTION 2			
Jog or high knees	10		
Stretch			
Hams			
Quads			
Calves			
30- to 40-second sprints, incline	Burnout		
OPTION 3			
Steady pace	30–40		
AB WORK (A.M.)	Reps	Weight	Reps Completed
Decline reverse rollup with Swiss ball	Burnout	N/A	
Decline reverse rollup with overhead jackknife	Burnout	N/A	
Weighted Owen crunch	Burnout		

DAY-6 EXERCISE LOG

SHOULDER AND LEG WORKOUT (P.M.)	Reps	Weight	Reps Completed
SUPERSET 1			
Dumbbell single-arm overhead press with a twist	8–10 (each arm)		
Squat	15–20		
REST			
SUPERSET 2			
Dumbbell single-arm overhead press with a twist	8–10 (each arm)		
Squat	15–20		
REST			
SUPERSET 3			
Dumbbell single-arm overhead press with a twist	8–10 (each arm)		
Squat	15–20		
REST			
T-bar row			
Set 1	12		
Set 2	12		
Set 3	12		
Walking lunge			
Set 1	15 (each leg)		
Set 2	15 (each leg)		
Set 3	15 (each leg)		
Bent-over (or seated) dumbbell rear delt raise			
Set 1	15		
Set 2	15		
Set 3	15		
Lying hamstring curl (or Romanian deadlift)			
Set 1	12–15		
Set 2	12–15		
Set 3	12–15		

The Exercises

DECLINE REVERSE ROLLUP WITH SWISS BALL

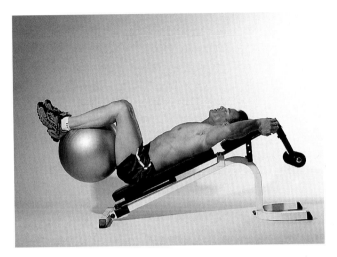
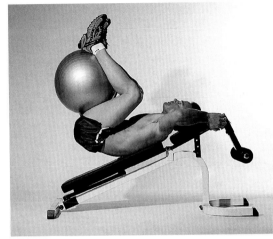

DECLINE REVERSE ROLLUP WITH OVERHEAD JACKKNIFE

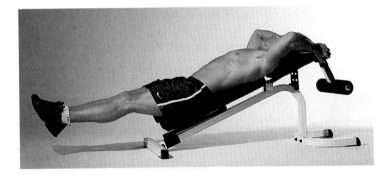

1 Lie head-highest on a decline bench, holding on to the leg pads or bench-end behind your head.

2 Roll your torso up by bringing your knees toward your forehead, letting your butt rise off the bench.

3 At the top of the movement, shoot your feet straight up in the air, straightening your legs and squeezing your abs. Then slowly roll your knees back toward your chest before lowering your trunk one vertebra at a time.

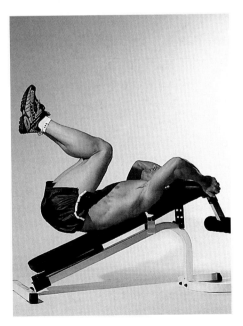
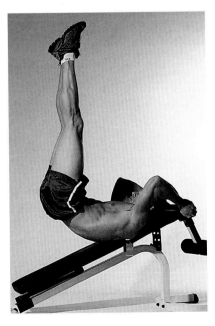

WEIGHTED OWEN CRUNCH

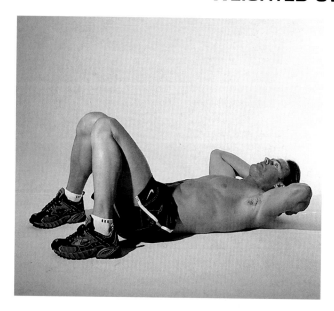 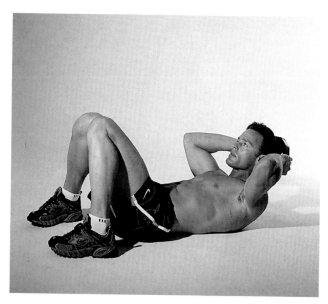

DUMBBELL SINGLE-ARM OVERHEAD PRESS
WITH A TWIST

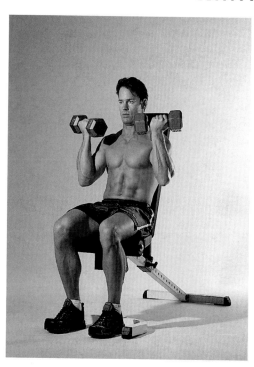 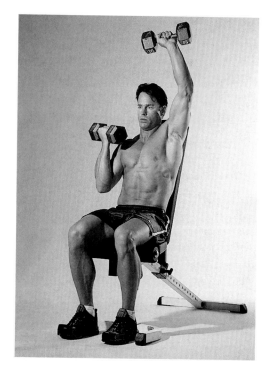

SQUAT

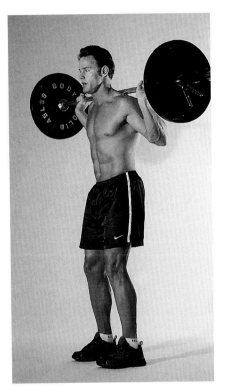 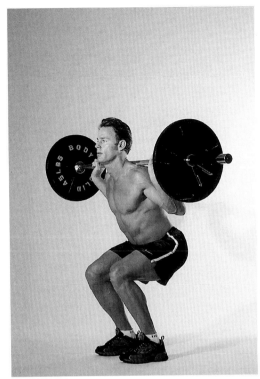

T-BAR ROW

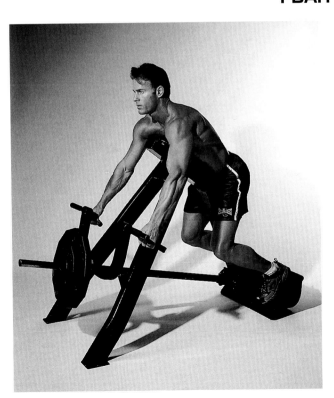 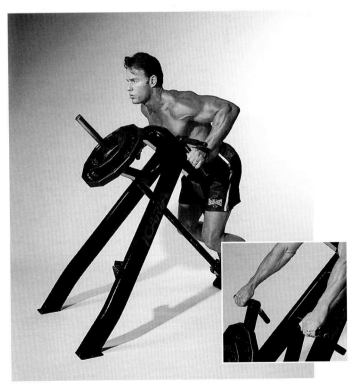

WALKING LUNGE

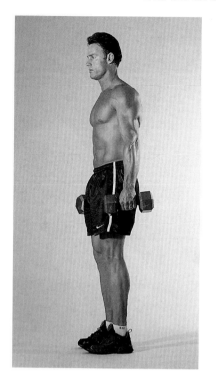
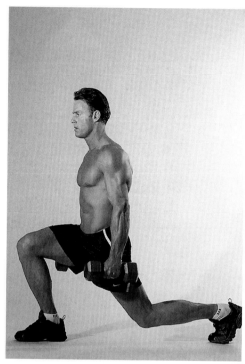

BENT-OVER DUMBBELL REAR DELT RAISE

1 Stand bent over like a down-hill skier, holding two light dumbbells straight down, with your palms facing your knees and your elbows just slightly bent.

2 Lift the weights out to the sides and slightly behind you until your upper arms are at shoulder level.

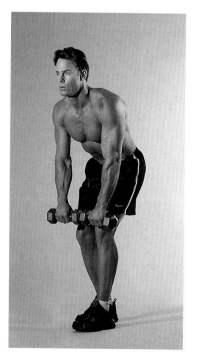
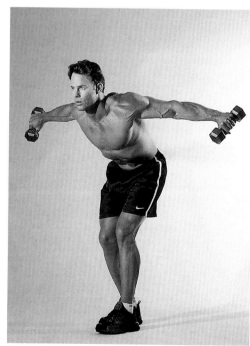

SEATED DUMBBELL REAR DELT RAISE

1 Sit at the side edge of a small bench, feet together, holding two light dumbbells behind your calves with your palms facing behind you.

2 Retract your back and keep your elbows slightly bent as you lift the weights back and out to the sides until your forearms are at shoulder level.

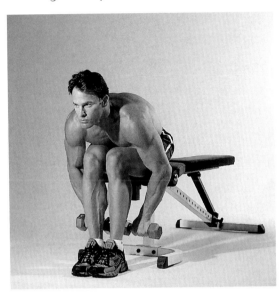 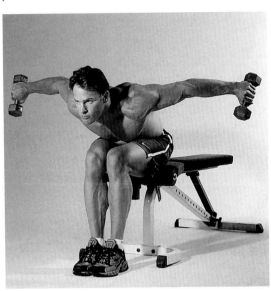

LYING HAMSTRING CURL

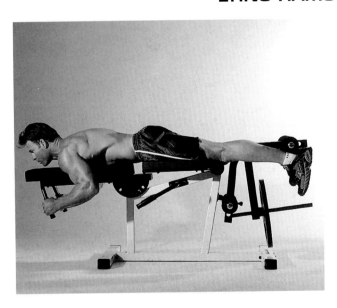 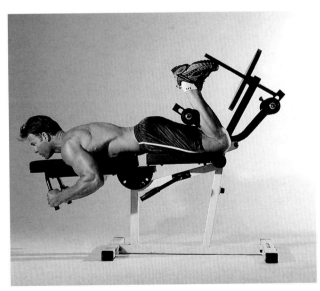

ROMANIAN DEADLIFT

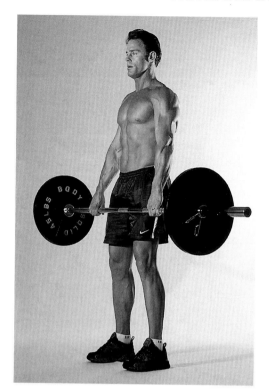 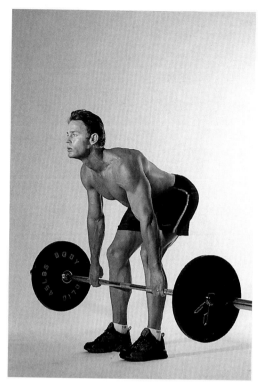

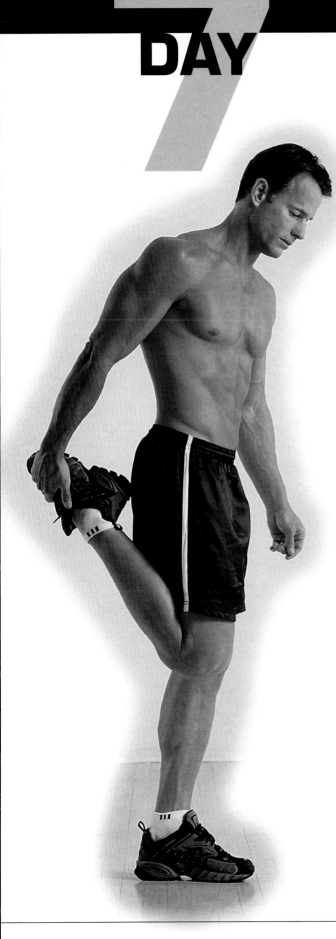

DAY 7

Congratulations! When you climb into bed tonight, you'll be halfway to the promised land.

Be proud of yourself. You've worked your butt off with relentless cardio sprinting and interval training, rigorous resistance training with vicious burnout sets, and a very strict diet. You've also put up with soreness that probably still hasn't gone away.

You've earned yourself a couple of breaks. Today I'm going to nix your weight workout. Let's give those muscles a chance to recover. And, what the hell, no ab work either!

Nevertheless, there's no such thing as a day off during the 2-Week Tweak. Your big gig is only a week away, so you need to make every day count. That's why, today, you're going to do double cardio: one workout in the A.M. and another in the P.M.

Work hard on that second cardio session! Picture the fat melting off your body, revealing the muscled results of all your hard work.

All in all, today is very unusual, yet profitable. You won't have much of a workout log, since there are no ab or weight exercises. And you won't eat anything today that you haven't eaten before, so we'll skip the "Kitchen Tactics" as well.

Here's what you still have to do.

6:00 A.M.

Wake-Up Call

Keep your daily cuppa joe, black, and your 8 ounces of water.

6:15 A.M.

Cardio

Do 30 to 40 minutes at a good, steady pace that keeps your heart rate up but allows you to have a conversation as you go (even if there's nobody to talk to). Follow up with stretches of all your upper- and lower-body muscle groups. Even though you aren't sprinting today, you're getting ready for lots of it in the days ahead. Stretches help.

7:30 A.M.

Breakfast

You should recognize these choices: scrambled egg whites with vegetables, hot oat bran, or a protein smoothie. If you don't have the ingredients memorized yet, turn back to pages 198 and 217. And slurp 12 ounces of water, of course.

10:00 A.M.

Mid-Morning Mini-Meal

The familiar protein bar you've grown to love, and the even more familiar 12 ounces of water.

12:30 P.M.

Lunch

Any of the previous lunches from this first week will be fine. They're on pages 196, 206, 216, 224, and 238.

3:00 P.M.

Mid-Afternoon Mini-Meal

Just like yesterday, suck back a soy milk–less, fruit-free protein smoothie. Chase it with 12 ounces of water.

5:30 P.M.

Pre-Workout Snack

Today your snack is prior to a cardio workout, not a weight session. So make it an apple for fructose fuel.

6:00 P.M.

Cardio

As in your morning cardio, do a 30- to 40-minute steady-pace haul.

Here's the twist (you knew one was coming, didn't you?): If you've been performing the same mode of cardio exercise every day, I want you to switch. For example, if you always use a stationary bike at the gym, try a treadmill. Or mix it up with several of them. Say, do 10 minutes on the bike, 10 minutes on the stairclimber, 10 minutes on the treadmill, and 10 on a ski machine.

One more option: If you're finding your groove on the treadmill, try different styles. Run backward for 2 minutes, or do a sideways shuffle for 2 minutes on each side. You can even try skipping. The point is to throw your body a curve.

7:30 P.M.

Dinner

Any of the previous dinner choices (from pages 196, 207, 216, 225, and 239) will work tonight. Like Old Faithful, there will be 12 ounces of water.

DAY-7 EXERCISE LOG

CARDIO (A.M.)	Min	Mode	Min Completed
Steady pace	30–40		
Upper- and lower-body stretches			

CARDIO (P.M.)	Min	Mode	Min Completed
OPTION 1			
Steady pace, different mode	30–40		
OPTION 2			
Steady pace, mixed machines			
Machine 1	10		
Machine 2	10		
Machine 3	10		
Machine 4	10		
OPTION 3			
Treadmill, steady pace, mixed styles	30–40		

"Never forget that your potential is more important than your problems."

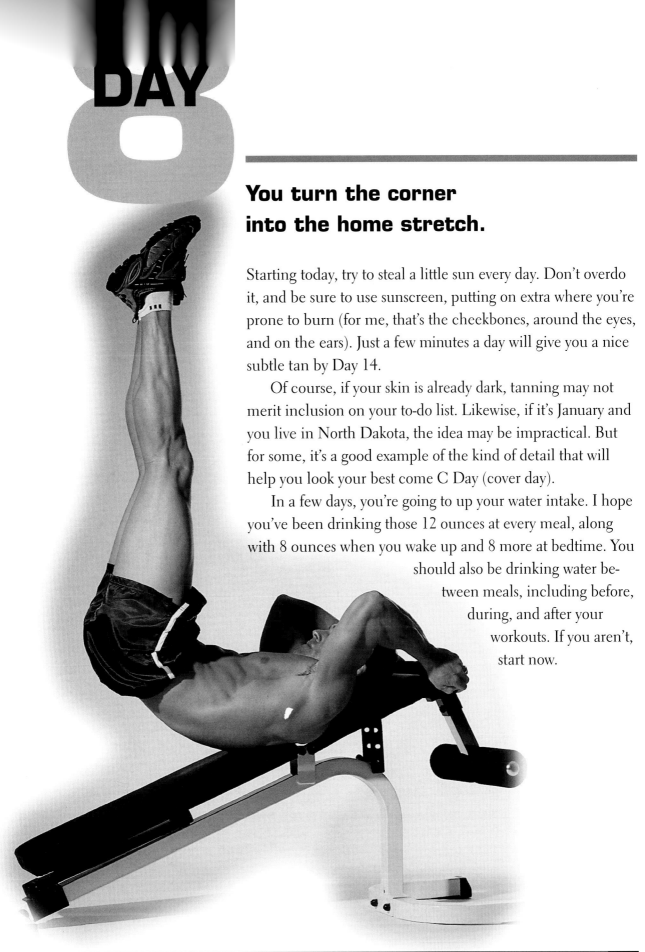

DAY 8

You turn the corner into the home stretch.

Starting today, try to steal a little sun every day. Don't overdo it, and be sure to use sunscreen, putting on extra where you're prone to burn (for me, that's the cheekbones, around the eyes, and on the ears). Just a few minutes a day will give you a nice subtle tan by Day 14.

Of course, if your skin is already dark, tanning may not merit inclusion on your to-do list. Likewise, if it's January and you live in North Dakota, the idea may be impractical. But for some, it's a good example of the kind of detail that will help you look your best come C Day (cover day).

In a few days, you're going to up your water intake. I hope you've been drinking those 12 ounces at every meal, along with 8 ounces when you wake up and 8 more at bedtime. You should also be drinking water between meals, including before, during, and after your workouts. If you aren't, start now.

Wake-Up Call

After your 8 ounces of water, trade in your black coffee for a double espresso. You'll need the extra caffeine when you get to the cardio. . . .

6:15 A.M.

Cardio

You're going to take it up a notch today, so get yourself into attack mode. I want every fiber of your being focused on one goal: kicking ass for 40 minutes.

There's no looking back now. If the treadmill is your cardio mode, crank up the incline. Don't hold on with your hands. Use your arms and rotate your trunk as you walk or jog. Pretend you're a piston powering one of those gnarly old black locomotives up a steep hill.

If you're on the stationary bike, take four-time Tour de France champion Lance Armstrong's advice: "Pound down on the pedals." Bravely program some added resistance into your ride. Don't hold back.

If you're doing 20-minute interval training indoors, show the rest of the early birds at the gym how fiercely you're driven. Do the same run/walk intervals as before but crank up the incline on the treadmill or the resistance on the bike.

Whatever you do, follow it up with a thorough stretching routine.

7:15 A.M.

Ab Work

Today, do two exercises that you're already familiar with.

→ Decline reverse rollup with overhead jack-knife: three sets of 20 reps

→ Side jackknife: two sets of 20 to 30 reps, each side

7:30 A.M.

Breakfast

Again, choose one of the three basic breakfasts (see pages 198 and 217 — if you pick oat bran, remember to use only ¼ banana). Drink 12 ounces of water. Yeah, I know, there's a lot of same-old, same-old in your meal choices. I've tried to include variety, but the top priority is the diminishing-carb, high-protein strategy. Believe me, it's worth it. And it's only for another 7 days.

10:00 A.M.

Mid-Morning Mini-Meal

Consume your standard protein bar and 12 ounces of water.

12:30 P.M.

Lunch

Pick any one of the lunch options (on pages 196, 206, 216, 224, and 238), with 12 ounces of agua.

3:00 P.M.

Mid-Afternoon Mini-Meal

Protein smoothie, made with whey powder, water, and peanut butter only. Drink 12 ounces of water.

5:30 P.M.

Pre-Workout Snack

Scarf down an apple or a small chicken breast, with 12 ounces of water.

6:00 P.M.

Workout

Today it's your back and your bi's, featuring lots of my favorite exercise: pullups. This workout is grueling. Start with three sets to burnout of each of the three pullup variations you've been doing: wide-grip, close-grip, and underhand-grip.

Then go to the lat-pulldown machine and start there with wide-grip lat pulldowns. Do three sets with descending rep counts, from 18 to 14 to 12. Follow with three sets of the close-grip version, with the rep count descending from 14 to 12 to 10.

Next come T-bar rows. Do four sets of 20 reps each, alternating between the palms-facing grip and the palms-down grip. Drop your poundage a bit with each set, but keep the between-set rest to a bare minimum.

Finish up with a pyramid giant set of dumbbell hammer curls. Here's how it works: Start with dumbbells that you can curl for 18 reps but that aren't so heavy you can't go on after those 18. Let's say they're 30 pounds. After the 18 reps, drop those dumbbells, grab a slightly lighter pair (say, 25 pounds), and do 16 reps. Drop those, pick up even lighter weights (maybe 20 pounds), and do 14. Keep dropping weight and reducing your number of reps by 2 until you do 8 reps at a very light weight. Then start back up the rep ladder again, moving up to 10 reps to 12 to 14 to 16 and topping out at 18 (if you make it that far), using heavier weights each set.

7:30 P.M.

Dinner

Your dinner du jour is any one of those you've enjoyed so far. (The menus du previous jours are on pages 196, 207, 216, 225, and 239.) Drink your obligatory 12 ounces of water with it.

DAY-8 EXERCISE LOG

CARDIO (A.M.)	Min	Mode	Min Completed
OPTION 1			
Steady pace, incline	40		
OPTION 2			
Steady pace	15–20		
Intervals, incline	20		
STRETCH			

AB WORK (A.M.)	Reps	Reps Completed	
Decline reverse rollup with overhead jackknife			
Set 1	20		
Set 2	20		
Set 3	20		
Side jackknife			
Set 1	20–30 (each side)		
Set 2	20–30 (each side)		

DAY-8 EXERCISE LOG

BACK AND BICEPS WORKOUT (P.M.)	Reps	Weight	Reps Completed
Wide-grip pullup			
Set 1	Burnout		
Set 2	Burnout		
Set 3	Burnout		
Close-grip pullup			
Set 1	Burnout		
Set 2	Burnout		
Set 3	Burnout		
Underhand pullup (chinup)			
Set 1	Burnout		
Set 2	Burnout		
Set 3	Burnout		
Wide-grip lat pulldown			
Set 1	18		
Set 2	14		
Set 3	12		
Close-grip lat pulldown with palms facing each other			
Set 1	14		
Set 2	12		
Set 3	10		
T-bar row			
Set 1 (palms facing)	20		
Set 2 (palms down, drop)	20		
Set 3 (palms facing, drop)	20		
Set 4 (palms down, drop)	20		
Dumbbell hammer curl			
Set 1	18		
Set 2 (drop)	16		
Set 3 (drop)	14		
Set 4 (drop)	12		
Set 5 (drop)	10		
Set 6 (drop)	8		
Set 7 (drop)	10		
Set 8 (drop)	12		
Set 9 (drop)	14		
Set 10 (drop)	16		
Set 11 (drop)	Burnout–18		

The Exercises

DECLINE REVERSE ROLLUP WITH OVERHEAD JACKKNIFE

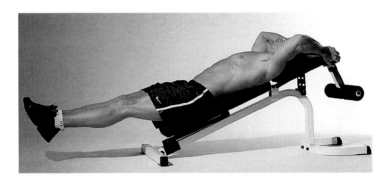

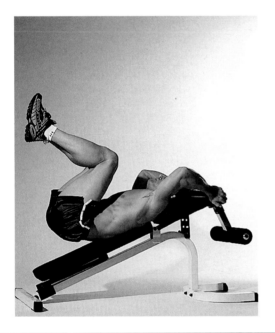

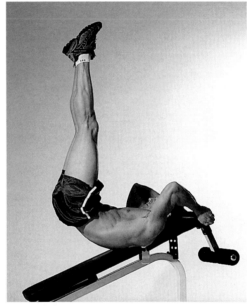

SIDE JACKKNIFE

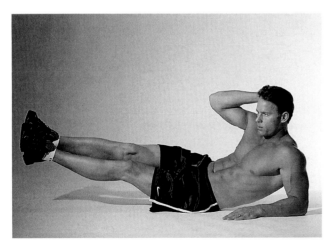

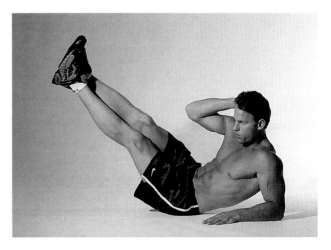

WIDE-GRIP PULLUP

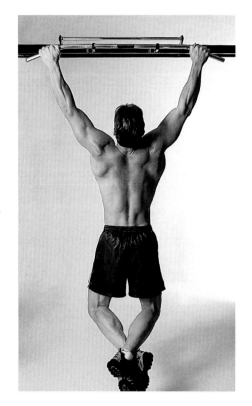 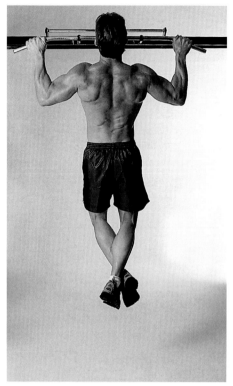

CLOSE-GRIP PULLUP

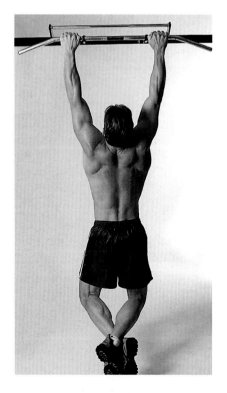 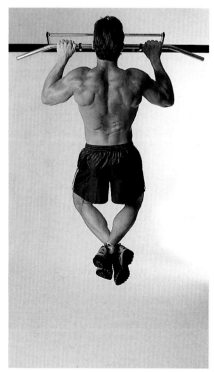

UNDERHAND PULLUP (CHINUP)

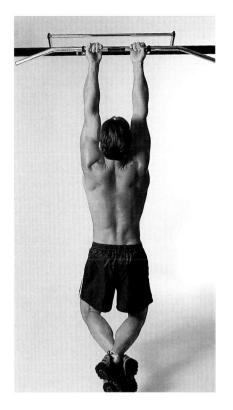 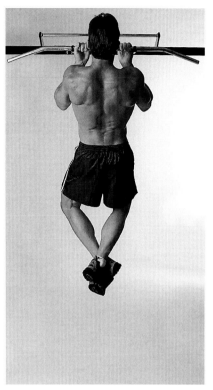

WIDE-GRIP LAT PULLDOWN

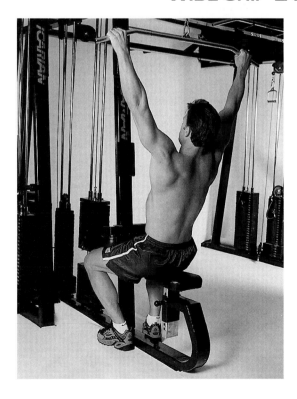 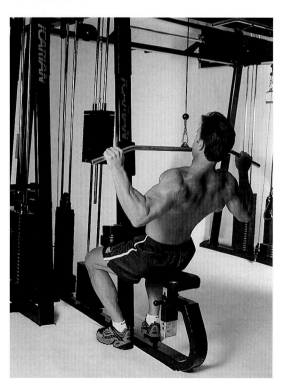

CLOSE-GRIP LAT PULLDOWN WITH PALMS FACING EACH OTHER

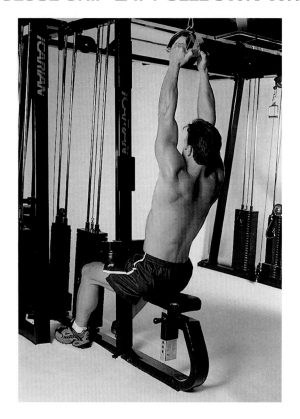
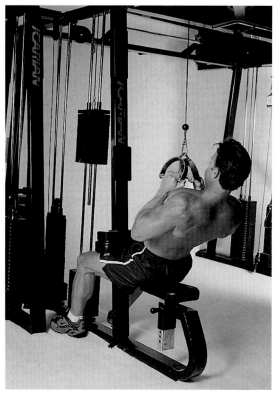

T-BAR ROW

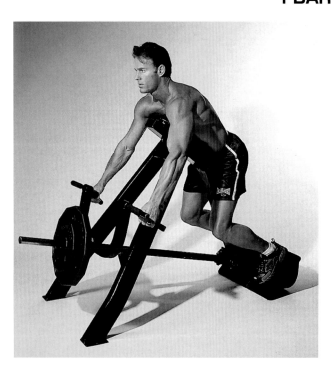
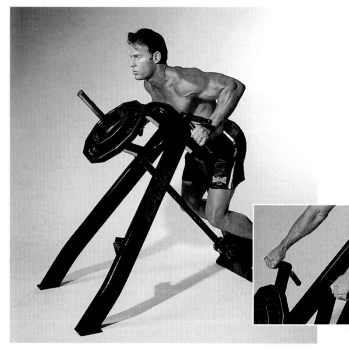

DUMBBELL HAMMER CURL

1 Stand holding two dumbbells at your outer thighs, palms facing each other.

2 Keep your palms facing each other as you curl the weights up to your shoulders. Pause, then slowly lower to the starting position.

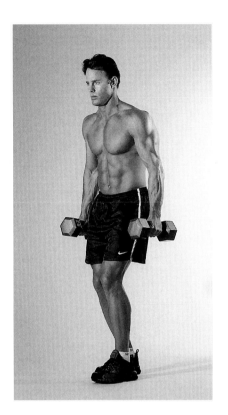

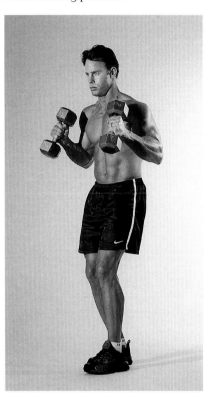

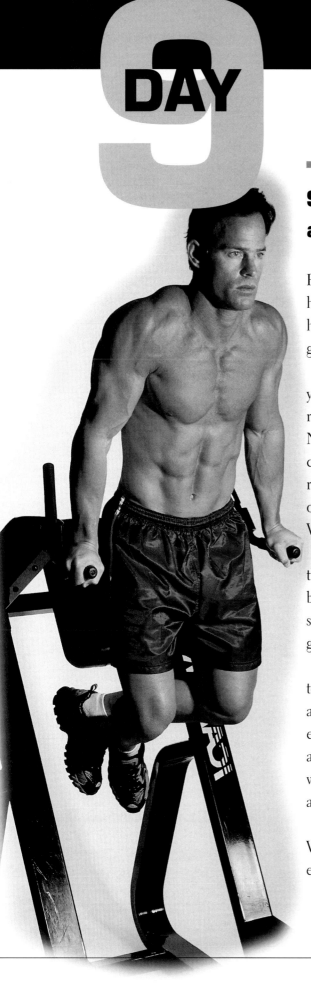

Starting to hate me a little bit right about now?

Remember, I'm just trying to bring out your best. If you hate me anyway, express it by dominating the workouts I have planned for you today. Show me up! As long as you get it done, I'm happy.

After completing that vicious back-and-bi's workout yesterday, you're probably having a hard time just reaching over your head and straightening out your arms. Not to mention how sore your calves and butt are from churning uphill for 40 minutes. You did do 40 minutes, right? Unless you're doing sprints or intervals, 40 minutes of morning cardio is mandatory at this point of your 2-Week Tweak.

Actually, I never doubted for a minute that you did those 40 minutes yesterday. Why should I? You've already blown your own mind with your willingness to eat large servings of raw pain. And in just 6 more days, you're going to blow everyone else's mind as well.

The Tweak only gets more intense now. You're going to drastically reduce your carbs and cut down on calories as well. Your smoothies are devoid of soy milk and fruit, even in the mornings. Your ½-cup servings of oat bran and brown rice dwindle down to ¼ cup each. Your pre-weight-lifting apple turns into a half-apple—or better yet, a protein alternative.

Yeah, I know what you're thinking: "Half an apple? Who eats half an apple? McKibbin has gone off the deep end!" Maybe so. But I know what works. So let's rock.

6:00 A.M.

Wake-Up Call

Quaff a double espresso and 8 ounces of water.

6:15 A.M.

Cardio

Start with 10 minutes of warmup: a walk, an easy jog, or a light ride on the bike. Then it's 20 minutes of sprinting—not full-on 100 percent sprinting for 20 seconds, but sprinting nonetheless. This is not simply an option; it's for everybody. Sprint at about 75 percent of full effort for 2 minutes. Then walk for a minute. Repeat that cycle (2-minute sprint, 1-minute walk) for 20 minutes. Be sure to stretch afterward.

7:00 A.M.

Ab Work

Perform relatively light ab work today. In fact, do the same routine as on Day 1 (back on page 196). That is, do three sets of Owen crunches at 25 reps apiece, and three sets of reverse rollups, also at 25 reps apiece.

7:30 A.M.

Breakfast

Select any of the breakfast options (they're still on pages 198 and 217). Put no fruit or soy milk in the smoothie; make it with water. If you choose oat bran, make it ¼ cup. Skip the toast with your egg whites. Now and forevermore, drink 12 ounces of pure water with your breakfast.

10:00 A.M.

Mid-Morning Mini-Meal

Reach for yet another protein bar and 12 ounces of water.

12:30 P.M.

Lunch

Prepare any of those trusty lunch options from pages 196, 206, 216, 224, and 238. If you include rice at all, make it ¼ cup. Drink 12 ounces of water.

3:00 P.M.

Mid-Afternoon Mini-Meal

It's the return of the protein smoothie—full of water, but fruit-less. Drain 12 ounces of water.

5:00/5:30 P.M.

Pre-Workout Snack

Halve an apple and eat one piece, or make a small chicken breast as directed on page 198. Starting today, you may have a pre-workout cup of coffee (no cream, no sugar) to give yourself a little kick start before you hit the weights.

6:00 P.M.

Workout

Today targets your chest and tri's, big time. The lineup of exercises looks like this.

→ Dumbbell bench press: three sets of 20 to 25 reps

→ Dip: three sets of 12 to 15 reps

→ Incline dumbbell bench press: two sets of 15 reps

→ Decline dumbbell bench press: two sets of 15 reps

→ Pec deck: three sets of 25 reps

→ Rope triceps pushdown: three sets of 25 reps

→ Lying triceps kickback: one set of 100 reps

Yeah, you read that last line right: 100 reps. Here's how you manage that. Get out six pairs of dumbbells (12, 10, 8, 6, 5, and 3 pounds). Do as many lying triceps kickbacks as you can with the two 12-pound weights. Then, without resting, go to the 10-pounders until burnout. Then grab the 8s, and so on until you hit 100 reps. Make that 100th repetition really count. On that last rep, hold the weights in the locked-out position for 30 seconds. This will give your triceps an unbelievable pump as well as create an intense isometric contraction in your upper back and shoulders.

7:30 P.M.

Dinner

Order from our established dinner menu (pages 196, 207, 216, 225, and 239), with tons of water.

DAY-9 WORKOUT LOG

CARDIO (A.M.)	Min	Mode	Min Completed
Easy pace	10		
Sprint (75% full effort)	2		
Walk	1	Walk	
Sprint (75% full effort)	2		
Walk	1	Walk	
Sprint (75% full effort)	2		
Walk	1	Walk	
Sprint (75% full effort)	2		
Walk	1	Walk	
Sprint (75% full effort)	2		
Walk	1	Walk	
Sprint (75% full effort)	2		
Walk	1	Walk	
Sprint (75% full effort)	2		
Stretch			

AB WORK (A.M.)	Reps	Reps Completed
Owen crunch		
Set 1	25	
Set 2	25	
Set 3	25	
Reverse rollup		
Set 1	25	
Set 2	25	
Set 3	25	

DAY-9 WORKOUT LOG

CHEST AND TRICEPS WORKOUT (P.M.)	Reps	Weight	Reps Completed
Dumbbell bench press			
Set 1	20–25		
Set 2	20–25		
Set 3	20–25		
Dip			
Set 1	12–15		
Set 2	12–15		
Set 3	12–15		
Incline dumbbell bench press			
Set 1	15		
Set 2	15		
Decline dumbbell bench press			
Set 1	15		
Set 2	15		
Pec deck			
Set 1	25		
Set 2	25		
Set 3	25		
Rope triceps pushdown			
Set 1	25		
Set 2	25		
Set 3	25		
Lying triceps kickback			
100-rep set	Burnout	12	
	Burnout	10	
	Burnout	8	
	Burnout	6	
	Burnout	5	
	Burnout	3 (30-sec final lockout)	

The Exercises

OWEN CRUNCH

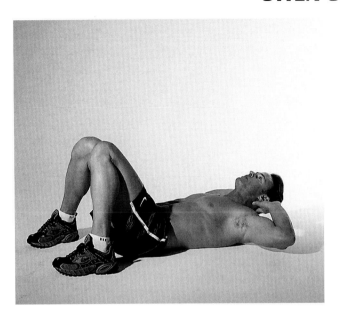
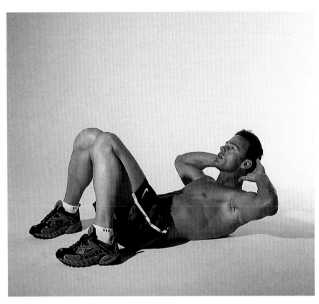

REVERSE ROLLUP

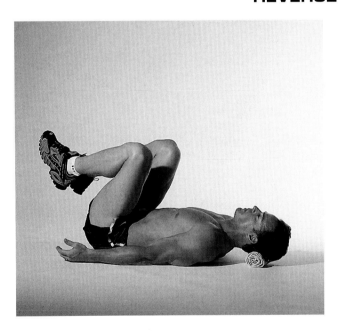
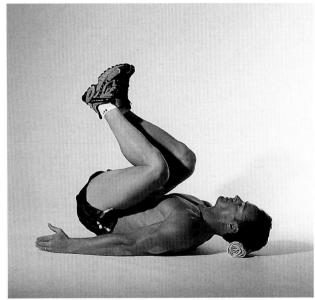

DUMBBELL BENCH PRESS

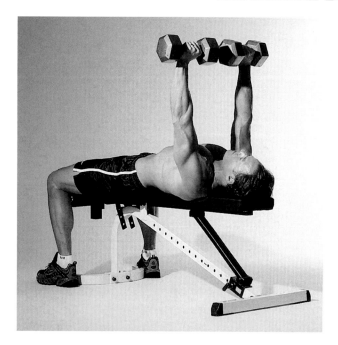
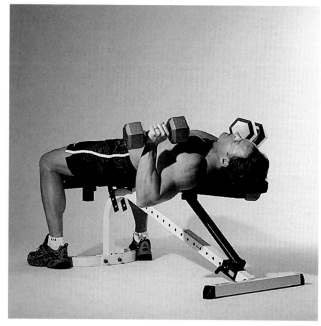

DIP

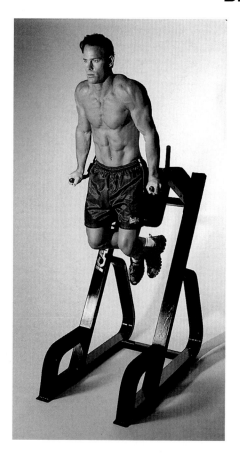
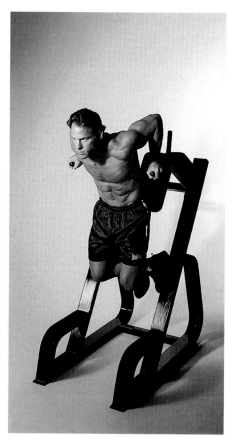

INCLINE DUMBBELL BENCH PRESS

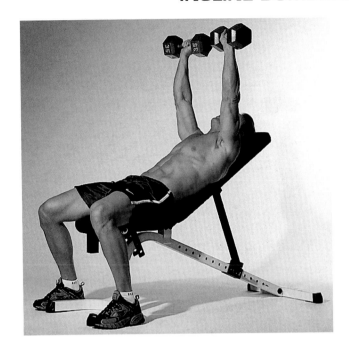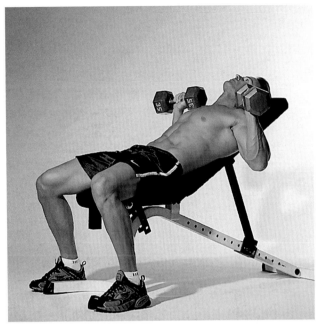

DECLINE DUMBBELL BENCH PRESS

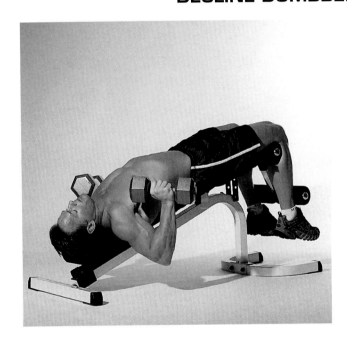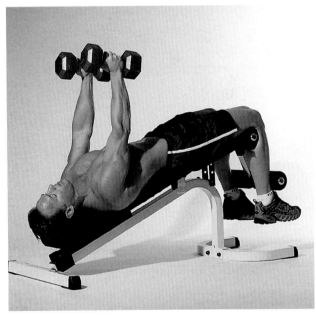

PEC DECK

1 Sit on the bench of the pec-deck machine with your feet flat and the seat adjusted so your elbows are just below shoulder-level as you place your forearms against the backs of the pads.

2 Use your chest muscles to bring your arms around in front of your body until the pads almost touch in front of you. Pause, then let the weights back slowly until they're in line with your torso. Don't use your hands to complete the contraction.

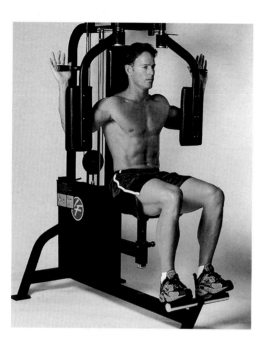 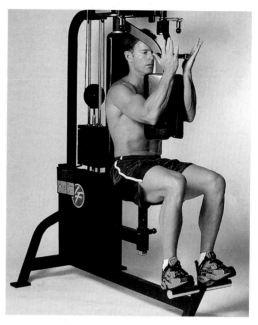

ROPE TRICEPS PUSHDOWN

1 Attach a rope handle to the high pulley of a cable station and grab it so your palms face each other. Start with your elbows bent 90 degrees and your upper arms against your sides.

2 Straighten your arms, allowing your hands to pull the rope ends outward at the bottom. Pause, then slowly return to the starting position.

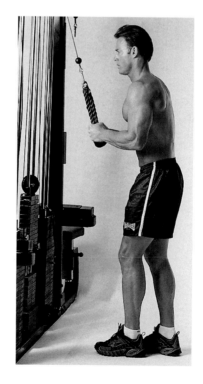 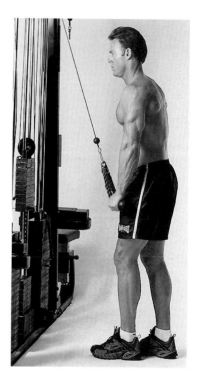

LYING TRICEPS KICKBACK

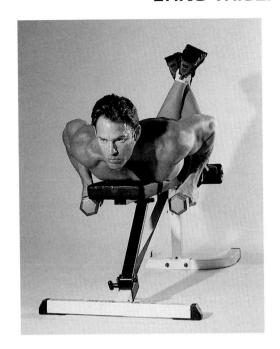 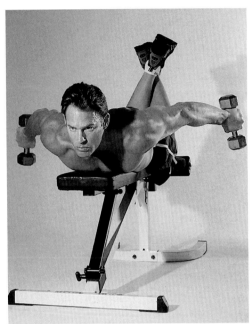

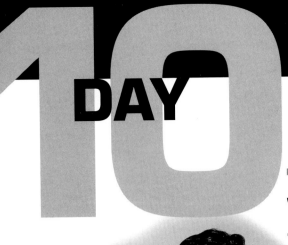

DAY 10

When you're working hard to peak out for a special day, you do some strange things.

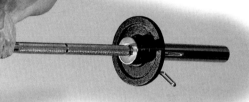

Today, I'm going to suggest one of the strangest. Starting 5 days before a scheduled cover shoot, I drink all my coffee through a straw. You should do the same if you think your brightest smile will make a difference. For me, it definitely does.

Believe me, I know how weird it is to sip espresso with a straw. But it's the only way to keep the java from staining your teeth.

Your other option is to 86 the coffee altogether—which is no option at all as far as I'm concerned. The straw thing is worth it; those extra-white pearlies will make a big difference come C Day.

Here's a reason to show off those choppers right now: no ab work today.

6:00 A.M.
Wake-Up Call

Look as macho as possible while sucking up a double espresso through a straw. You can lose the prop when it's time for your 8 ounces of water.

6:15 A.M.
Cardio

And now for something completely different: Go full-time on a cardio machine or activity that you've never done—or that you only tried for 10 minutes on Day 7. You know that strange machine you always glance at as you walk by in the gym? Maybe you're not even sure what it is; they're getting pretty creative in the aerobic hardware industry these days. Anyway, what the hell, give it a try. Lick your chops, get the kinks out of your neck, shake your arms, and then make that machine wish it had never been built. There's a new machine king in the gym now: you! Dominate that thing for 40 hard-core minutes. Follow it up with a stretch session.

7:30 A.M.
Breakfast

Start getting strict and skimpy. Today you can break your fast with a protein smoothie, made with water (no soy milk) and 1 tablespoon of peanut butter (as well as the protein powder, of course). But no fruit. If you'd rather chew, have the scrambled egg whites, with onions, tomatoes, and spinach. But no toast. And forget about the oat bran from now on. Don't dare forget about the 12 ounces of water.

10:00 A.M.
Mid-Morning Mini-Meal

All hail the mighty protein bar and 12 ounces of water.

12:30 P.M.
Lunch

Round up one of your customary lunches (they haven't moved from pages 196, 206, 216, 224, and 238), but without any brown rice.

3:00 P.M.
Mid-Afternoon Mini-Meal

It's the same as today's first breakfast option: another water-and-peanut-butter-and-protein-powder smoothie.

5:00/5:30 P.M.
Pre-Workout Snack

Repeat yesterday's apple half or chicken breast. Or there's a third option (hooray!) that you'll have from now on: half of a small can of white albacore tuna, packed in water. You don't need bread or mayonnaise. Just rinse the tuna and eat it. Coffee is optional.

6:00 P.M.
Workout

It's time for another shoulder workout. Start off with alternating dumbbell single-arm overhead presses with a twist. Do two sets with each arm, 20 reps each set (press with one arm and then press with the other until you've done 20 presses with each, counting one-one, two-two, and so on).

Then do drop sets of side lateral raises, as follows. Choose two dumbbells with which you can just barely do 15 repetitions. As soon as you finish those 15 reps, grab lighter dumbbells and do a set of 25. Repeat the heavy set of 15 and the lighter 25.

Next, do two supersets of dumbbell single-arm rear deltoid raises with standing upright rows (the latter is one of the few straight-bar lifts in the Tweak). Do a set of 20 delt raises with each arm, followed immediately by a set of 15 to 20 rows. Then, after minimal rest, repeat that superset.

Dinner
Get used to the following two choices, which are basically double portions of your pre-workout snack options with vegetables added. They'll be your steady dinner companions from now until C Day. Choice one is two chicken breasts, seasoned with olive or flaxseed oil (1 tablespoon), balsamic vinegar, fresh lemon juice, and pepper. Choice 2 is a can of white albacore tuna, rinsed and drained, sans bread, mayo, or other sandwich fixins. Either can be accompanied by a cup of spinach, broccoli, or asparagus, with the same oil-vinegar-lemon-pepper seasoning.

DAY-10 EXERCISE LOG

CARDIO (A.M.)	Min	Mode	Min Completed
Steady pace, new machine	40		
Stretch			

SHOULDER WORKOUT (P.M.)	Reps	Weight	Reps Completed
Alternating dumbbell single-arm overhead press with a twist			
Set 1	20 (each arm)		
Set 2	20 (each arm)		
Side lateral raise			
Set 1	15		
Set 2 (drop)	25		
Set 3 (add)	15		
Set 4 (drop)	25		
SUPERSET 1			
Dumbbell single-arm rear deltoid raise	20 (each arm)		
Standing upright row	15–20		
SUPERSET 2			
Dumbbell single-arm rear deltoid raise	20		
Standing upright row	15–20		

The Exercises

ALTERNATING DUMBBELL SINGLE-ARM OVERHEAD PRESS WITH A TWIST

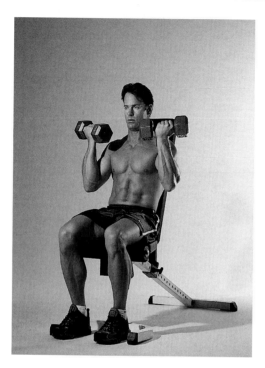
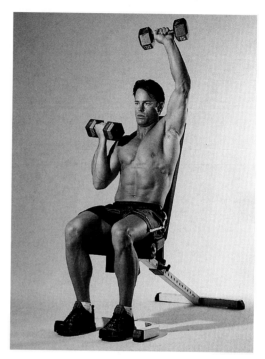

SIDE LATERAL RAISE

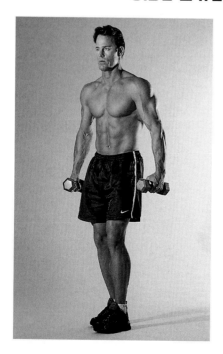
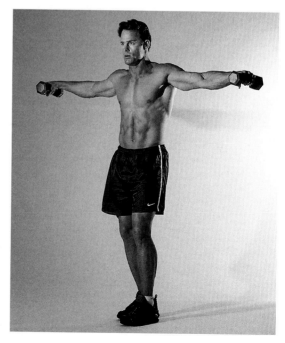

DUMBBELL SINGLE-ARM REAR DELTOID RAISE

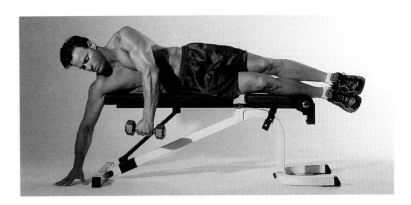

1 Grab a dumbbell with your nondominant hand (your left if you're right-handed). Lie on your dominant side on a bench, placing your free hand on the floor to brace yourself. Extend your working arm down toward the floor, with your elbow slightly bent and your palm facing you.

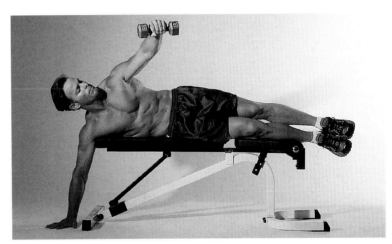

2 Keeping your elbow slightly bent, slowly lift the weight until your arm is slightly above shoulder level. Pause, then lower to the starting position. When you finish your reps, move to the other end of the bench and do the same number of reps with your other arm.

STANDING UPRIGHT ROW

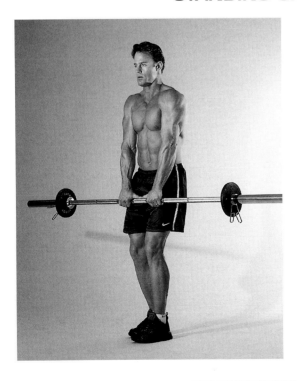

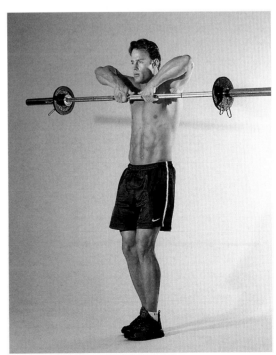

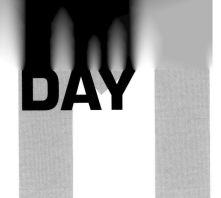

DAY 11

How's your energy level? If it's down a bit, there's a good reason.

You've cut your calories, and you've eliminated dry carbs—pasta and potatoes from the get-go, and now bread and rice. You're still getting carbs in the vegetables you're eating, though.

Your protein intake is going up. And the more protein you eat, the more water you need to drink as well. So as of today, adjust your water dose at each meal from 12 ounces to 16 ounces, or about two typical glasses. Increase to 10 ounces before your morning coffee and 10 before bed, putting you at 116 ounces a day. Try to add at least 16 more ounces on your own somewhere.

Because you're consuming fewer overall calories and no dry carbs at all, you're going to shorten your workouts. You're also going to make them more intense. Now, I know exactly what you're thinking: "You're telling me that what I've been doing hasn't been intense? What's your idea of intense, McKibbin?" You're about to find out.

A tip for today: If you have hair on your back or anyplace else where it's not considered cool for whatever you'll be doing on the big day, now's the time for a wax job. If you get it done today, you'll have 72 hours to clear up if your skin breaks out in reaction to the waxing. You may or may not consider this stuff a priority, but I do. With the kind of body shots I do—and the hirsute back I have—it's gotta be done.

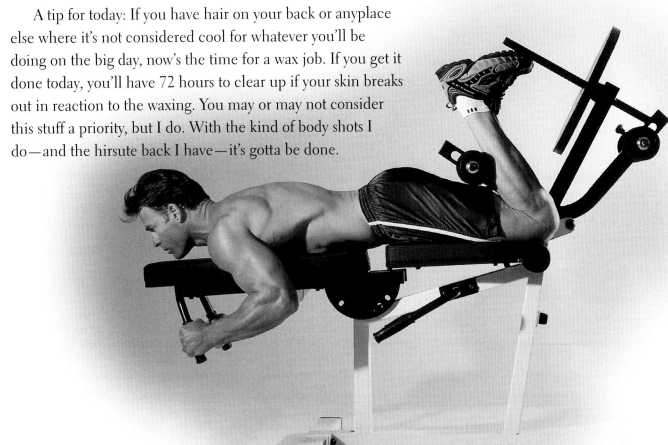

6:00 A.M.
Wake-Up Call
You still need that straw, but you can go back to regular black coffee if you want. I prefer espresso. Either way, drink 10 to 12 ounces of water.

6:15 A.M.
Cardio
Start with a 5-minute warmup and some light stretching. Then give me 20 minutes of interval training, as follows: Do a 2-minute-on/1-minute-off routine. For the first of those 2 "on" minutes, run at 60 to 70 percent of full effort. Take it up to 80 to 90 percent for the second minute. At the end of the 2 minutes, drop down to a walk. This is your time to breathe deeply and recover. When that minute is up, start the cycle again. Keep it up for 20 minutes—that is, for six or seven cycles.

By shortening the duration of your cardio work and increasing the intensity, you jack up your metabolism even more, turning yourself into a testosterone mountain, a fat-burning volcano.

6:45 A.M.
Ab Work
Do just two sets today: one set of reverse rollups to burnout followed by a set of Owen crunches, also to burnout. Stretch afterward.

7:30 A.M.
Breakfast
This meal is the same as yesterday. (Look back at page 280 if you need a reminder of your options.) Drink 16 ounces of water.

10:00 A.M.
Mid-Morning Mini-Meal
Welcome back your usual protein bar and 16 ounces of water.

12:30 P.M.
Lunch
Strip down any of the lunch options (pages 196, 206, 216, 224, and 238) until they're devoid of brown rice and bread. You need a little fat, so if you don't use a tablespoon of olive or flaxseed oil, have a little bit of avocado (about 2 table-spoonfuls). Imbibe those 16 ounces of water.

3:00 P.M.
Mid-Afternoon Mini-Meal
Have a protein smoothie, a protein bar, a half-can of white albacore tuna, or one chicken breast. Belt back 16 more ounces of water.

5:00/5:30 P.M.
Pre-Workout Snack
Go back to page 280 and eat what it says there.

6:00 P.M.
Workout
It's a back-and-legs day. Do this workout almost like circuit training, taking little or no rest between sets and exercises. You've done all these exercises before.

→ Wide-grip lat pulldown: two drop sets at 20 and 15 reps. In other words, do a set of 20 reps with the heaviest possible weight, then immediately do 15 reps at a lower weight

→ Squat: one set of 25 to 30 reps

→ Close-grip lat pulldown with palms facing each other: two drop sets at 20 and 15 reps

→ Walking lunge (but unlike in the photo, do not use weights today): one set to burnout

→ T-bar row: four drop sets, each set at 20 reps (using a lower weight each time)

→ Lying hamstring curl: one set to burnout, which should be at least 30 reps

7:30 P.M.
Dinner
Your options are the same as last night (page 281), but down a full 16 ounces of water.

DAY-11 EXERCISE LOG

CARDIO (A.M.)	Min	Mode	Min Completed
Easy-pace warmup	5		
Stretch			
Interval-Cycle 1			
60–70% full effort	1		
80–90% full effort	1		
Easy pace or walk	1		
Interval-Cycle 2			
60–70% full effort	1		
80–90% full effort	1		
Easy pace or walk	1		
Interval-Cycle 3			
60–70% full effort	1		
80–90% full effort	1		
Easy pace or walk	1		
Interval-Cycle 4			
60–70% full effort	1		
80–90% full effort	1		
Easy pace or walk	1		
Interval-Cycle 5			
60–70% full effort	1		
80–90% full effort	1		
Easy pace or walk	1		
Interval-Cycle 6			
60–70% full effort	1		
80–90% full effort	1		
Easy pace or walk	1		
Interval-Cycle 7			
60–70% full effort	1		
80–90% full effort	1		
Easy pace or walk	1		

DAY-11 EXERCISE LOG

AB WORK (A.M.)	Reps	Reps Completed	
Reverse rollup	Burnout		
Owen crunch	Burnout		
Stretch			

BACK AND LEGS WORKOUT (P.M.)	Reps	Weight	Reps Completed
Wide-grip lat pulldown			
Set 1	20		
Set 2 (drop)	15		
Squat	25–30		
Close-grip lat pulldown with palms facing each other			
Set 1	20		
Set 2 (drop)	15		
Walking lunge	Burnout	N/A	
T-bar row			
Set 1	20		
Set 2 (drop)	20		
Set 3 (drop)	20		
Set 4 (drop)	20		
Lying hamstring curl	Burnout (30+)		

"I don't think I'm being naive when I say that the lessons you learn by getting and staying fit translate to all other pursuits."

The Exercises

REVERSE ROLLUP

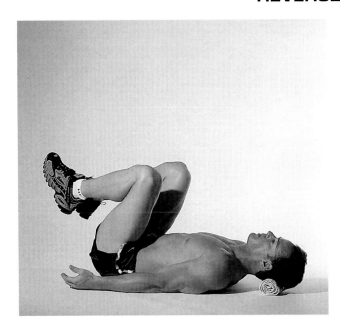 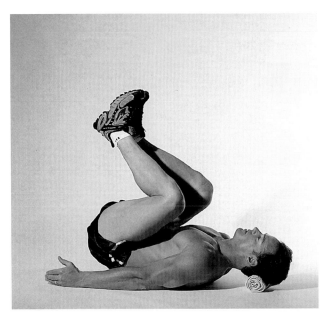

OWEN CRUNCH

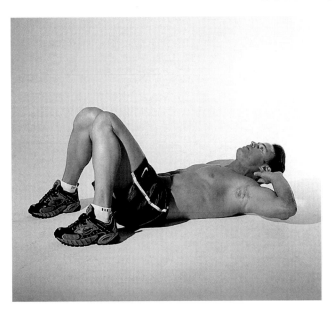 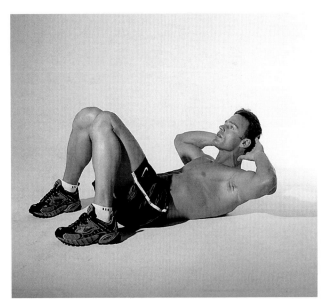

WIDE-GRIP LAT PULLDOWN

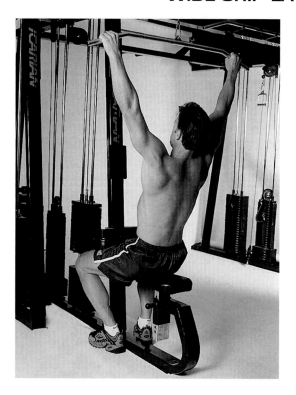 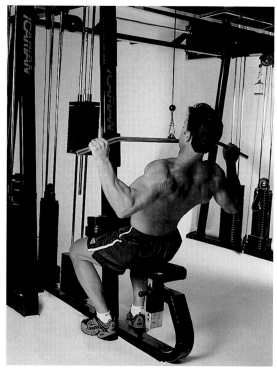

SQUAT

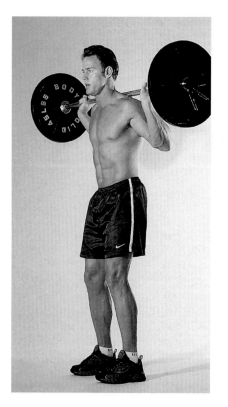 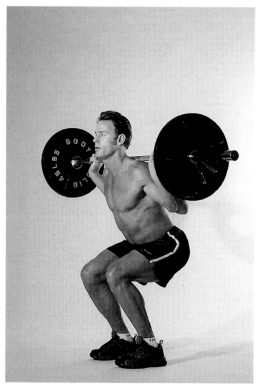

CLOSE-GRIP LAT PULLDOWN WITH PALMS FACING EACH OTHER

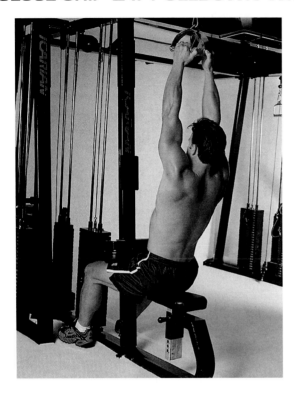
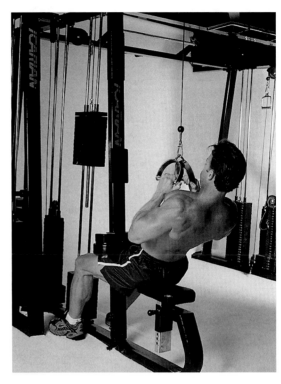

WALKING LUNGE

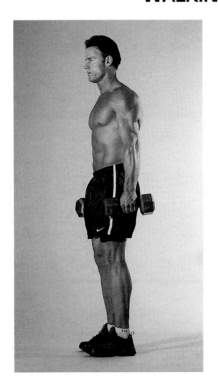
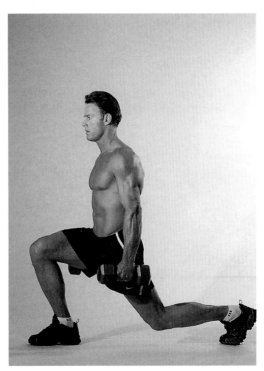

T-BAR ROW

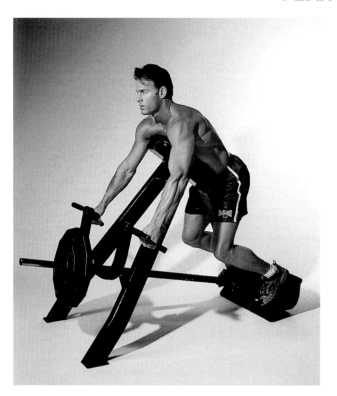
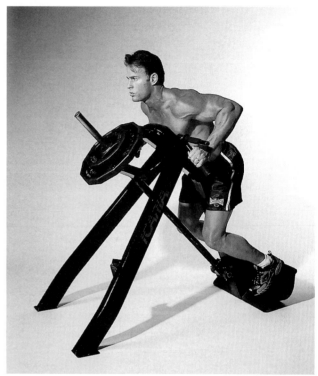

LYING HAMSTRING CURL

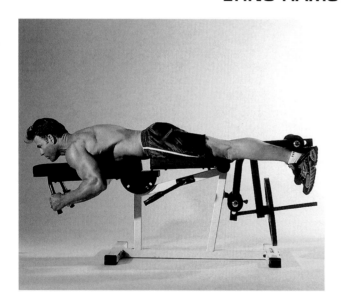
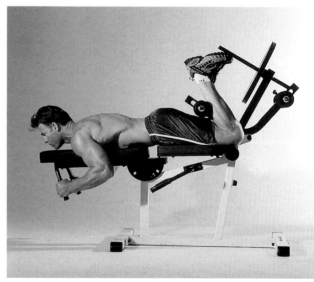

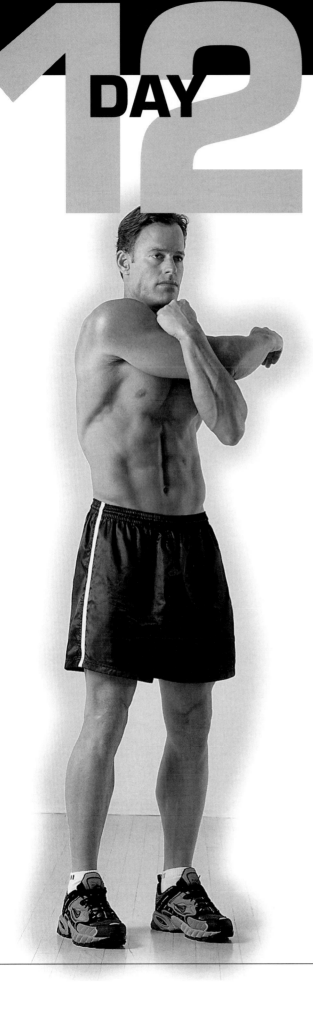

DAY 12

Three more days and you da man.

You've come this far, so eating just a little more pain is no problem, is it? And by now, you're truly an animal. You want more.

So guess what? You're actually going to get less. And for good reason. I've broken you down one way or another every single day for 11 days now, so you're taking a day off from all lifting as well as from ab work. And no extra cardio either!

Take advantage by eating dinner earlier and getting some extra shut-eye tonight. Or just relax.

Don't worry, this day off from strength training will not set you back. Truth is, it's just what you need right now. Trust me, it will do your body a world of good. And besides, you've definitely earned it.

Today's tip: My wife turned me on to this strategy that I rejected out of hand at first. Eventually I broke down and ended up liking the results. Here's the deal: When I get a lot of sun, it tends to bleach out my eyelashes. So now I get them professionally darkened at a hair salon. Yeah, it sounds a little weird, but it pays off in front of the camera. If you're going to do it, make sure you get it done today. For the first 24 hours or so, it looks a little too much like makeup. After that, though, it gives you one more subtle little improvement for the big day.

6:00 A.M.
Wake-Up Call
Swallow coffee and 10 to 12 ounces of water.

6:15 A.M.
Cardio
Cool the intensity a bit today. Just get on the bike or treadmill and give me 40 fast, crisp, steady minutes. I like to set the program on manual, put it on level 10 or 12, and keep the RPMs hovering around 100. I recommend listening to some hard-core heavy metal, or whatever rocks your boat. Get your stretching in afterward.

7:30 A.M.
Breakfast
It's still the same as the past 2 days (see page 280). Remember, toast is a thing of the past at this point. So is the fruit and soy milk in your smoothie. Be sure to use a tablespoon of olive oil or flaxseed oil to cook your egg whites. You need that fat. Wash it down with 16 ounces of water.

10:00 A.M.
Mid-Morning Mini-Meal
Opt for your usual protein bar and 16 ounces of water, or a water-based protein smoothie with no soy milk and no fruit—in other words, just water, whey protein, and 1 tablespoon of peanut butter.

12:30 P.M.
Lunch
As with breakfast, the alternatives are the same as yesterday (page 286). Swallow 16 ounces of water.

3:00 P.M.
Mid-Afternoon Mini-Meal
You guessed it—same as yesterday: a protein smoothie or bar, or a half-can of white albacore tuna, or one small chicken breast, all moistened with 16 more ounces of water.

5:00/5:30 P.M.
Pre-Workout Snack
This is an elective today, of course, since you're not doing a workout. If you'd like a snack about now, though, choose from the same options first proposed on Day 10 (page 280).

6:30/7:00 P.M.
Dinner
As I said, have dinner a little earlier tonight, and use the extra time for rest, rest, and more rest. Your dinner choices are the same as the previous 2 days (see page 281). Remember, you're allowed no dry carbs of any kind—just chicken or albacore tuna, and vegetables. You know your beverage: 16 ounces of water.

DAY-12 EXERCISE LOG

CARDIO (A.M.)	Min	Mode	Min Completed
Steady pace	40		
Stretch			

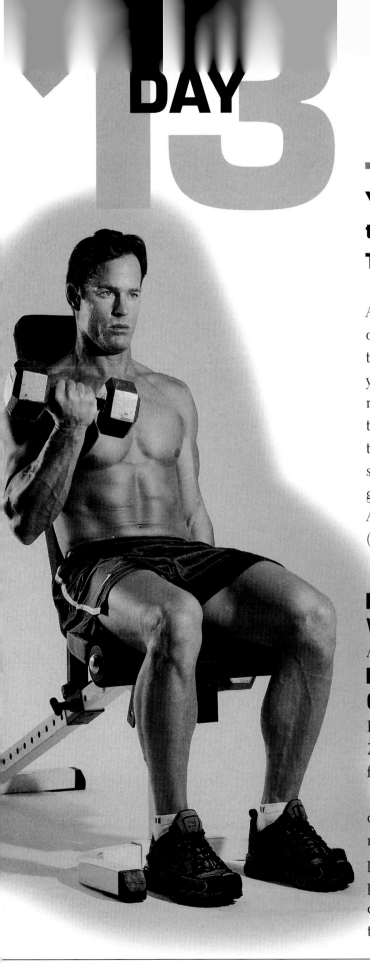

DAY 13

You're getting down to the wire now. Time for some strategy.

As you know, you've totally deprived your system of dry carbs for the past few days. At the same time, your body is storing very little water between your muscles and your skin. Today, you're going to reintroduce some clean dry carbs into your body to soak up any remaining water. That will have the effect of making your muscles stand out. Also, since dry carbs have a high sugar index, they'll give you more energy for your big day tomorrow. And that extra sugar will bring out your vascularity (visible veins over your newly ripped body).

Skip the six-pack–specific stuff again today.

6:00 A.M.
Wake-Up Call
Arise to coffee and 12 ounces of water.

6:15 A.M.
Cardio
Repeat either the Day-11 interval routine (page 286) or the mellower straight-ahead workout from yesterday (page 294).

I would do the interval program, with its balls-out sprinting. I like the way it focuses every inch of my physical and mental being. It also gives me a psychological edge as the 2-Week Tweak nears completion. Think about it: How many other dudes are doing this psycho stuff? Not many. That can make the difference between you and the rest of the pack.

But don't let me pressure you. The Day-12 program is fine. It's your call. One suggestion, though: If you have the energy to think about it for more than a minute, choose the intervals.

Whichever you go with, stretch afterward.

7:30 A.M.
Breakfast
The debate over which came first—the smoothie or the egg whites—continues. There's no contest about the 16 ounces of water.

10:00 A.M.
Mid-Morning Mini-Meal
Have protein in bar or smoothie form. And there's 16 ounces of water, water, everywhere.

12:30 P.M.
Lunch
Don't tell me you're tired of our beloved lunch specials—or the 16 ounces of you-know-what.

3:00 P.M.
Mid-Afternoon Mini-Meal
It's déjà vu about a protein smoothie, a protein bar, a half-can of white tuna, or a chicken breast (not to mention a 16-ounce glass of water).

5:00/5:30 P.M.
Pre-Workout Snack
Unlike yesterday, this isn't optional today. But your choices are still the same ones from page 280.

6:00 P.M.
Workout
Today you aim at your arms. You haven't before focused exclusively on them on any one day, so today we'll shock them to life.

This session is supersetted, with a triceps movement immediately followed (without rest) by a biceps move. Repeat three times.

→ The first pair are 20 reps of standing triceps pushdowns and 15 to 20 reps of seated dumbbell curls with palms out.

→ Next are 20 reverse-grip triceps pulldowns (use less weight than with the regular, over-hand-grip triceps pushdowns), followed by alternating seated dumbbell curls with a twist for 15 reps with each arm.

→ The final superset consists of rope triceps pushdowns (25 reps; remember the flare at the end) and dumbbell hammer curls (15 reps). In case you're wondering, I prefer dumbbells for all curl exercises because they allow a more natural range of motion in your arms, wrists, and elbows.

7:30 P.M.
Dinner
Supper is the same as yesterday with one key addition. Tonight, have half of a baked potato without butter, sour cream, or any other topping. Just eat the spud.

KITCHEN TACTICS

Baked Potato
Russet potatoes, with thick, dark skin, bake best.

→ Preheat the oven to 425°F.

→ Rinse and dry a potato.

→ Jab it with a fork a few times.

→ Rub some olive oil on it.

→ Wrap the potato in aluminum foil.

→ Bake for about 45 minutes, or until a knife goes through easily.

You may want to bake two potatoes at once, if you're going to want the optional tater portions in tomorrow's mid-morning snack and lunch, on the final day of the Tweak.

DAY-13 EXERCISE LOG

CARDIO (A.M.)	Min	Mode	Min Completed
OPTION 1			
Easy-pace warmup	5		
Stretch			
Interval-Cycle 1			
60–70% full effort	1		
80–90% full effort	1		
Easy pace or walk	1		
Interval-Cycle 2			
60–70% full effort	1		
80–90% full effort	1		
Easy pace or walk	1		
Interval-Cycle 3			
60–70% full effort	1		
80–90% full effort	1		
Easy pace or walk	1		
Interval-Cycle 4			
60–70% full effort	1		
80–90% full effort	1		
Easy pace or walk	1		
Interval-Cycle 5			
60–70% full effort	1		
80–90% full effort	1		
Easy pace or walk	1		
Interval-Cycle 6			
60–70% full effort	1		
80–90% full effort	1		
Easy pace or walk	1		
Interval-Cycle 7			
60–70% full effort	1		
80–90% full effort	1		
Easy pace or walk	1		
OPTION 2			
Steady pace	40		
STRETCH			

DAY-13 EXERCISE LOG

ARMS WORKOUT (P.M.)	Reps	Weight	Reps Completed
SUPERSET 1A			
Standing triceps pushdown	20		
Seated dumbbell curl with palms out	15–20		
SUPERSET 1B			
Standing triceps pushdown	20		
Seated dumbbell curl with palms out	15–20		
SUPERSET 1C			
Standing triceps pushdown	20		
Seated dumbbell curl with palms out	15–20		
SUPERSET 2A			
Reverse-grip triceps pulldown	20		
Alternating seated dumbbell curl with a twist	15 (each arm)		
SUPERSET 2B			
Reverse-grip triceps pulldown	20		
Alternating seated dumbbell curl with a twist	15 (each arm)		
SUPERSET 2C			
Reverse-grip triceps pulldown	20		
Alternating seated dumbbell curl with a twist	15 (each arm)		
SUPERSET 3A			
Rope triceps pushdown	25		
Dumbbell hammer curl	15		
SUPERSET 3B			
Rope triceps pushdown	25		
Dumbbell hammer curl	15		
SUPERSET 3C			
Rope triceps pushdown	25		
Dumbbell hammer curl	15		

The Exercises

STANDING TRICEPS PUSHDOWN

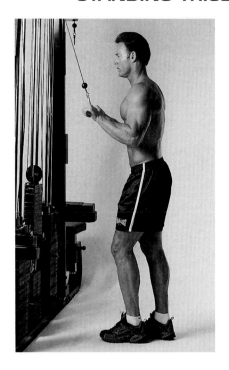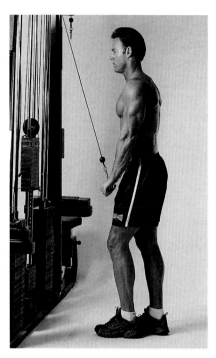

SEATED DUMBBELL CURL WITH PALMS OUT

1 Sit at the very end of a bench, holding two dumbbells below your outer thighs with overhand grips.

2 Moving only your forearms, curl the weights to your shoulders so your palms face away from you at the top of the movement. Then return to the starting position.

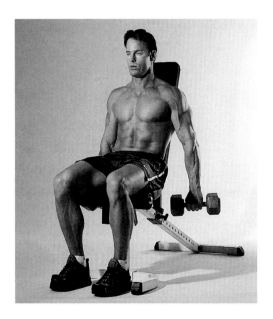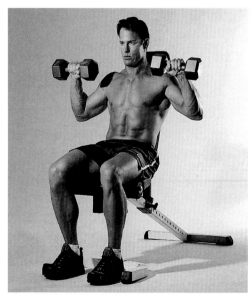

REVERSE-GRIP TRICEPS PULLDOWN

1 Attach the short, straight bar to the high pulley of a cable station. Stand as you would for a triceps pushdown, but grip the bar underhanded—that is, with your palms facing up.

2 Keep your elbows close to your sides as you move only your forearms to lower the bar to thigh level. Then return to the staring position.

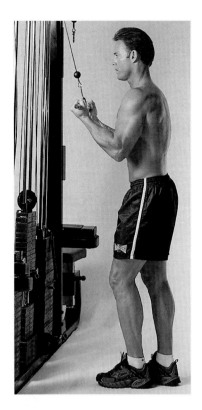
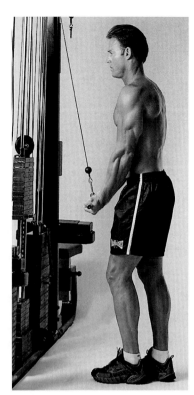

ALTERNATING SEATED DUMBBELL CURL WITH A TWIST

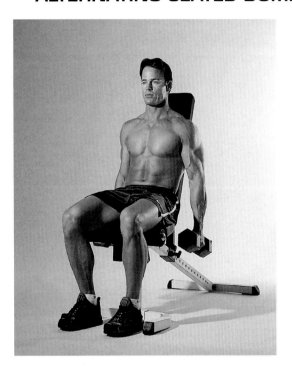
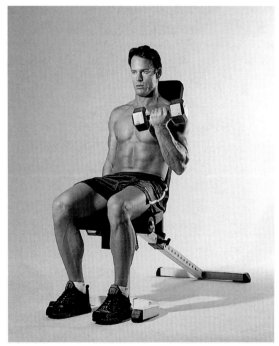

ROPE TRICEPS PUSHDOWN

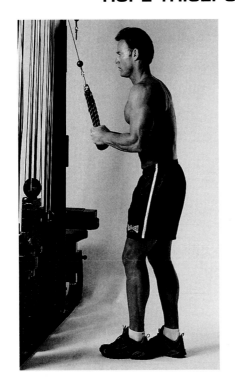
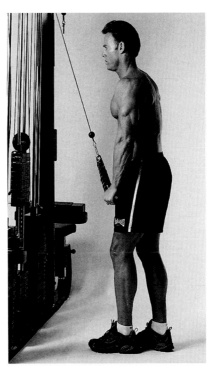

DUMBBELL HAMMER CURL

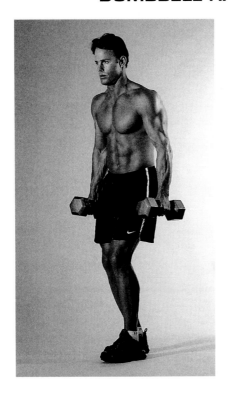
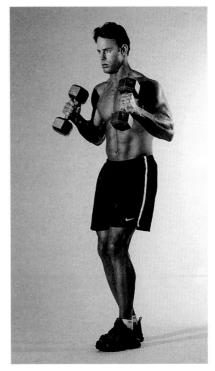

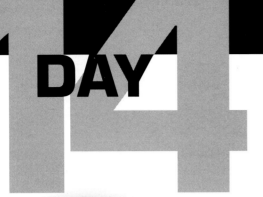

DAY 14

You are now the master of your own destiny.

You have all the power. You are physically and mentally disciplined. Your willpower to shun sweets and junk food has been unwavering. You've mastered cardio, resistance, and a strict nutrition regimen. You've transformed yourself into a lean, mean, fat-burning machine. You look great and you feel great.

Today is your day to shine. But unless you're going to party from sunup to sundown, you can still do a little something for your body today—a final tweak to hit your highest peak.

So I'm going to give you a day's routine. You won't do any evening weight workout, however, or any A.M. ab exercises. If you have to shift this schedule around to accommodate your big event, by all means do so. But don't blow off the day completely as far as exercise is concerned. The morning cardio will really help your energy for the day. And the morning eating strategy with the final dose of water-soaking dry carbs in the form of potato is very important.

One final eating tip: Start popping grapes at the exact time you want to peak and look your best. This will flush your system with sugar, highlighting your vascularity.

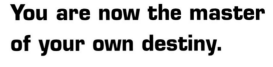

6:00 A.M.
Wake-Up Call
Have a pre-cardio caffeine boost and 8 ounces of water.

6:15 A.M.
Cardio
Just like yesterday, go for sprinting intervals or a steady-pace routine. Man, you should be flying! Don't forget the stretching afterward.

7:30 A.M.
Breakfast
Get your peaking protein with a smoothie or egg whites. Also eat the other half of that baked potato from last night. It will further soak up any water stored between your skin and muscles, emphasizing your cuts. Drink 12 ounces of water. (Don't worry, it won't replace what was just sucked up by the spud.)

10:00 A.M.
Mid-Morning Mini-Meal
In addition to your protein smoothie, protein bar, half-can of tuna fish, or chicken breast, you can have another ¼ baked potato. Also down 12 ounces of water.

12:30 P.M.
Lunch
You can add some brown rice, or even another half-potato, to one of the five meals you've been rotating: (1) chicken breast with green beans, asparagus, broccoli, or raw or steamed spinach; (2) fish and broccoli; (3) chicken or turkey salad; (4) lean red meat with spinach or edamame; or (5) chicken fajitas with black beans. Add 12 ounces of water.

3:00 P.M.
Mid-Afternoon Mini-Meal
Your snack stuff remains what it's been since Day 10 (page 280), with 12 ounces of water.

5:00/5:30 P.M.
Pre-Workout Snack
There's no workout to snack for. Still, you can have an apple or chicken breast, plus 12 ounces of water.

7:30 P.M.
Dinner
Splurge, dude. You deserve it.

Tomorrow, it's back to the regular version of the Cover Model Workout.

> *"It's never too late to find your niche, to begin something that feels right to you."*

DAY-14 EXERCISE LOG

CARDIO (A.M.)	Min	Mode	Min Completed
OPTION 1			
Easy-pace warmup	5		
Stretch			
Interval-Cycle 1			
60–70% full effort	1		
80–90% full effort	1		
Easy pace or walk	1		
Interval-Cycle 2			
60–70% full effort	1		
80–90% full effort	1		
Easy pace or walk	1		
Interval-Cycle 3			
60–70% full effort	1		
80–90% full effort	1		
Easy pace or walk	1		
Interval-Cycle 4			
60–70% full effort	1		
80–90% full effort	1		
Easy pace or walk	1		
Interval-Cycle 5			
60–70% full effort	1		
80–90% full effort	1		
Easy pace or walk	1		
Interval-Cycle 6			
60–70% full effort	1		
80–90% full effort	1		
Easy pace or walk	1		
Interval-Cycle 7			
60–70% full effort	1		
80–90% full effort	1		
Easy pace or walk	1		
OPTION 2			
Steady pace	40		
STRETCH			

PHOTO CREDITS

INDEX